# The Alpha Formula:

*The Ultimate Guide to Natural Testosterone Boosting for Men Over 40 at Peak Performance and Elevate Your Hormonal Health and Vitality*

## Lewis Finan

# Table of Contents

# **Introduction**:

Welcome to "The Alpha Formula: The Ultimate Guide to Natural Testosterone Boosting for Men Over 40 at Peak Performance and Elevate Your Hormonal Health and Vitality." In this comprehensive guide, we will delve into the world of testosterone and explore effective strategies to naturally enhance testosterone levels, enabling you to reclaim your youthful vitality and optimize your overall well-being.

As men age, testosterone levels gradually decline, leading to a myriad of physical and mental changes. Reduced energy, diminished muscle mass, increased body fat, decreased libido, and even mood swings are some of the common signs associated with declining testosterone. However, the good news is that by adopting natural approaches, we can reverse this decline and rejuvenate our hormonal health.

"The Alpha Formula" is specifically designed to empower men over 40 with the knowledge and tools necessary to boost testosterone production naturally. By understanding the intricate mechanisms of testosterone synthesis and exploring evidence-based techniques, you will be able to optimize your hormonal balance and unlock your full potential.

This guide will take you on a journey through various aspects of testosterone optimization, starting with an overview of the importance of testosterone in male health. We will then explore the factors that contribute to declining testosterone levels, including lifestyle choices, diet, exercise, sleep patterns, stress management, and environmental factors.

Throughout the chapters, you will discover a wide range of strategies and techniques to naturally elevate testosterone levels. We will discuss the benefits of specific exercises and strength training regimens that have been shown to stimulate testosterone production. Additionally, we will explore the role of nutrition and delve into the power of specific foods, vitamins, minerals, and supplements in promoting healthy testosterone levels.

Understanding the crucial connection between sleep, stress, and hormonal balance is another vital component of this guide. You will learn how to optimize your sleep patterns and implement stress reduction techniques to support optimal testosterone production and overall well-being.

"The Alpha Formula" also recognizes the importance of mindset and mental health in maintaining hormonal balance. We will delve into techniques to cultivate a positive mindset, manage stress, and create a supportive environment that contributes to your hormonal health and vitality.

Our guide is backed by the latest scientific research and incorporates expert advice from leading professionals in the field of men's health and hormonal optimization. Each chapter is meticulously crafted to provide you with practical, actionable steps that you can easily implement into your daily routine.

Whether you are looking to regain your youthful vigor, enhance your physical performance, or improve your overall well-being, "The Alpha Formula" is your comprehensive roadmap to achieving peak performance and elevating your hormonal health and vitality.

Get ready to embark on a transformative journey that will empower you to reclaim your alpha status and unlock the true potential that lies within. Let's dive in and discover the secrets to natural testosterone boosting for men over 40!

# Chapter 1: Understanding Testosterone

Testosterone is a hormone that plays a vital role in the development and maintenance of various physiological and psychological processes in both males and females. It is primarily known as the male sex hormone, but it is also present in females, albeit in smaller amounts. In this chapter, we will explore the functions, sources, regulation, and effects of testosterone in the human body.

**Functions of Testosterone**

Testosterone performs a range of functions in the body, influencing various aspects of physical and mental health. Here are some key functions:

## 1. Sexual Development and Reproduction:

During puberty, testosterone is responsible for the development of primary and secondary sexual characteristics in males. It stimulates the growth of the penis, testes, and scrotum, as well as the deepening of the voice and the growth of facial and body hair. In females, testosterone contributes to the development of the ovaries and helps regulate the menstrual cycle.

➢ *Muscle Mass and Bone Density:*

Testosterone plays a significant role in the development and maintenance of muscle mass and bone density. It promotes protein synthesis, which is essential for muscle growth, and helps prevent muscle wasting. Additionally, testosterone stimulates the production of red blood cells, aiding in oxygen transport and enhancing athletic performance.

➢ *Metabolism and Body Fat Distribution:*

Testosterone influences metabolism, promoting the burning of fat and helping to maintain a healthy body weight. It also affects body fat distribution, with higher testosterone levels typically associated with reduced abdominal fat.

➢ *Mood and Cognitive Function:*

Testosterone plays a role in mood regulation and cognitive function. Adequate testosterone levels contribute to a sense of well-being, motivation, and focus. Low testosterone levels have been associated with mood disorders, such as depression, and cognitive decline.

## 2. Sources and Regulation of Testosterone

The production and regulation of testosterone involve a complex interplay between various organs and hormones. Here's an overview of the process:

> ***Testes:***

The testes are the primary source of testosterone in males. Specialized cells called Leydig cells within the testes produce testosterone in response to luteinizing hormone (LH) secreted by the pituitary gland.

> ***Ovaries and Adrenal Glands:***

In females, the ovaries and adrenal glands are the primary sources of testosterone. The ovaries produce testosterone in small amounts, contributing to libido and overall well-being. The adrenal glands produce testosterone in both males and females, but it is a minor source compared to the testes or ovaries.

> ***Hypothalamus-Pituitary-Gonadal Axis:***

The hypothalamus and pituitary gland play a crucial role in regulating testosterone production. The hypothalamus secretes gonadotropin-releasing hormone (GnRH), which stimulates the pituitary gland to release LH and follicle-stimulating hormone (FSH). LH, in turn, stimulates the Leydig cells in the testes (or ovaries in females) to produce testosterone.

> *Feedback Mechanisms:*

Testosterone production is tightly regulated by a negative feedback mechanism. When testosterone levels are high, the hypothalamus and pituitary gland reduce the secretion of GnRH, LH, and FSH, which subsequently decreases testosterone production. Conversely, low testosterone levels trigger an increase in GnRH, LH, and FSH secretion to stimulate testosterone production.

## 3. Effects of Testosterone

Testosterone exerts various effects on different systems and functions in the body. Here are some notable effects:

> *Physical Effects:*

- Increased muscle mass and strength
- Improved bone density and reduced risk of osteoporosis
- Enhanced libido and sexual function
- Regulation of hair growth and balding patterns

> *Psychological Effects:*

- Improved mood and sense of well-being
- Increased motivation and drive

- Enhanced cognitive function, including memory and spatial abilities
- Influence on aggression and competitiveness

## ➤ *Health Effects:*

- Cardiovascular health: Testosterone helps maintain healthy cholesterol levels and promotes cardiovascular health.
- Metabolic health: Adequate testosterone levels are associated with improved insulin sensitivity and reduced risk of metabolic disorders such as diabetes.
- Red blood cell production: Testosterone stimulates the production of red blood cells, which is important for oxygen transport and overall health.
- Immune system function: Testosterone plays a role in modulating immune system activity and response.

Testosterone is a hormone with multifaceted functions and effects in the human body. It is crucial for sexual development, muscle mass, bone density, metabolism, mood regulation, cognitive function, and overall health. Understanding the functions, sources, regulations, and effects of testosterone provides valuable insights into the complexities of human physiology and the importance of hormonal balance. In the subsequent chapters, we will delve deeper into specific aspects of testosterone, including its role in different stages of life, the effects of testosterone imbalances, and the potential therapeutic applications of testosterone-related treatments.

**1.1 Introduction to Testosterone and Its Importance**

Testosterone is a hormone that plays a crucial role in the development and functioning of the human body. It is primarily known as the male sex hormone, but it is present in both males and females, albeit in different amounts. Testosterone is responsible for a wide range of physiological and psychological processes, making it an essential hormone for overall health and well-being. In this article, we will explore the importance of testosterone, its functions, and the effects of testosterone imbalances on the body.

## 1. What is Testosterone?

Testosterone belongs to a group of hormones known as androgens. It is produced primarily in the testes in males and in the ovaries and adrenal glands in females. Testosterone is also present in small quantities in the bloodstream of both sexes. During fetal development, testosterone plays a crucial role in the development of male genitalia and other male characteristics. In males, it continues to be produced throughout life, supporting various bodily functions.

## 2. Functions of Testosterone

Testosterone serves numerous functions in the body, influencing both physical and psychological aspects of human health. Here are some key functions of testosterone:

➤ *Sexual Development:*

During puberty, testosterone promotes the development of primary and secondary sexual characteristics in males. It stimulates the growth of the penis, testes, and scrotum, as well as the deepening of the voice and the growth of facial and body hair. In females, testosterone contributes to the development of the ovaries and helps regulate the menstrual cycle.

➤ *Muscle Mass and Strength:*

Testosterone plays a significant role in the development and maintenance of muscle mass and strength. It promotes protein synthesis, which is essential for muscle growth, and inhibits muscle breakdown. Higher testosterone levels are associated with increased muscle mass and improved athletic performance.

➤ *Bone Health:*

Testosterone is essential for maintaining healthy bones and preventing osteoporosis. It stimulates bone mineralization and helps maintain bone density. In cases of low testosterone levels, such as in older men or women experiencing hormonal changes during menopause, the risk of osteoporosis and fractures increases.

➤ *Metabolism and Body Fat:*

Testosterone influences metabolism, helping to regulate fat distribution and maintain a healthy body weight. It promotes the burning of fat, particularly in the abdominal region. Low testosterone levels are often associated with increased body fat and a higher risk of obesity.

> ***Libido and Sexual Function:***

Testosterone plays a vital role in sexual desire (libido) and sexual function in both males and females. It contributes to sexual arousal, supports erectile function in males, and enhances overall sexual satisfaction.

> **Mood and Well-being:**

Testosterone has an impact on mood regulation and overall well-being. Adequate testosterone levels are associated with a sense of vitality, motivation, and overall positive mood. Low testosterone levels have been linked to mood disorders such as depression and decreased quality of life.

> ***Cognitive Function:***

Testosterone also influences cognitive function, including memory, attention, and spatial abilities. It plays a role in maintaining cognitive health and may contribute to the prevention of cognitive decline and age-related neurodegenerative diseases.

## 3. Testosterone Imbalances and Effects

Imbalances in testosterone levels can have significant effects on the body and overall health. Both low and high levels of testosterone can lead to various symptoms and health issues:

### ➢ Low Testosterone (Hypogonadism):

Low testosterone levels, known as hypogonadism, can cause a range of symptoms, including:

- Decreased libido and sexual dysfunction
- Fatigue and decreased energy levels
- Loss of muscle mass and strength
- Increased body fat and weight gain
- Mood swings, irritability, and depression
- Reduced cognitive function and memory problems
- Decreased bone density2. High Testosterone (Hyperandrogenism):
- Elevated testosterone levels, known as hyperandrogenism, can also have adverse effects on the body, such as:
- Acne and oily skin
- Excessive facial and body hair growth (hirsutism)
- Male pattern baldness
- Menstrual irregularities and fertility issues in females
- Aggression and irritability
- Sleep disturbances
- Increased risk of cardiovascular diseases

It is important to note that testosterone imbalances can occur due to various factors, including natural hormonal fluctuations, medical conditions, medications, and lifestyle factors. If you suspect a testosterone imbalance, it is essential to consult with a healthcare professional for proper evaluation and management.

## 4. Maintaining Healthy Testosterone Levels

Maintaining healthy testosterone levels is crucial for overall health and well-being. While testosterone naturally declines with age, there are lifestyle choices that can help support healthy testosterone levels:

➢ ***Balanced Diet:***

Eating a nutritious and balanced diet is important for hormone production and overall health. Include foods rich in zinc, vitamin D, omega-3 fatty acids, and other essential nutrients. Examples include lean meats, fish, eggs, nuts, seeds, and leafy greens.

➢ ***Regular Exercise:***

Engaging in regular physical activity, including both cardiovascular exercises and strength training, can help optimize testosterone levels. Exercise promotes muscle growth, fat loss, and overall hormonal balance.

➢ *Adequate Sleep:*

Getting enough quality sleep is crucial for hormone regulation, including testosterone production. Aim for 7-8 hours of uninterrupted sleep each night.

➢ *Stress Management:*

Chronic stress can disrupt hormone balance, including testosterone levels. Engage in stress management techniques such as meditation, deep breathing exercises, yoga, or engaging in hobbies and activities you enjoy.

➢ *Weight Management:*

Maintaining a healthy weight is important for hormonal balance. Excess body fat, especially around the waist, can contribute to imbalances in testosterone levels.

➢ *Limit Alcohol and Substance Use:*

Excessive alcohol consumption and substance use can negatively impact testosterone production. Limiting or avoiding these substances can help maintain healthy hormone levels.

Testosterone is a vital hormone that plays a crucial role in numerous physiological and psychological processes in both males and females.

From sexual development and muscle mass to mood regulation and cognitive function, testosterone influences various aspects of human health. Understanding the functions of testosterone and the effects of imbalances is essential for maintaining overall well-being. By adopting a healthy lifestyle and seeking appropriate medical care when needed, individuals can support healthy testosterone levels and optimize their health and quality of life.

## 1.2 How Testosterone Levels Change with Age

Testosterone is a hormone that plays a vital role in the development and maintenance of various physiological processes in the human body. As individuals age, there is a natural decline in testosterone levels, which can have significant effects on overall health and well-being. In this article, we will explore how testosterone levels change with age, the factors that contribute to this decline, and the potential implications for health and quality of life.

### 1. Testosterone Levels during Development and Young Adulthood

During fetal development and throughout puberty, testosterone levels increase significantly, leading to the development of primary and secondary sexual characteristics. In males, testosterone levels surge during puberty, resulting in the growth of the penis, testes, and scrotum, as well as the deepening of the voice and the growth of facial and body hair. In females, testosterone levels also rise, contributing to the development of the ovaries and regulating the menstrual cycle.

During young adulthood (late teens to early twenties), testosterone levels reach their peak. This period is characterized by optimal testosterone production, supporting muscle development, bone density, sexual function, and overall vitality.

## 2. Age-Related Decline in Testosterone Levels

Starting in the late twenties or early thirties, testosterone levels gradually decline with age. This decline is a normal part of the aging process and is often referred to as "andropause" or "late-onset hypogonadism" in men. While the decline is gradual, the rate of decline can vary among individuals. On average, testosterone levels decrease by approximately 1% per year after the age of 30.

Several factors contribute to the age-related decline in testosterone levels:

➤ *Leydig Cell Function:*

Leydig cells, which are responsible for testosterone production in the testes, may become less efficient with age. This can result in decreased testosterone synthesis and secretion.

➤ *Hypothalamic-Pituitary-Gonadal (HPG) Axis:*

The HPG axis, which regulates testosterone production, may experience changes with age. The hypothalamus and pituitary gland may become less sensitive to hormonal signals, leading to decreased secretion of gonadotropin-releasing hormone (GnRH), luteinizing hormone (LH), and follicle-stimulating hormone (FSH). This reduced stimulation of the Leydig cells ultimately results in lower testosterone production.

> *Testicular Changes:*

Age-related structural and functional changes in the testes can also contribute to decreased testosterone production. These changes may include a decline in the number and size of Leydig cells, reduced testicular blood flow, and alterations in testicular tissue.

> *Increased Binding of Testosterone:*

As individuals age, there may be an increase in the production of sex hormone-binding globulin (SHBG), a protein that binds to testosterone in the bloodstream. When testosterone binds to SHBG, it becomes less available for use by the body's tissues, leading to lower levels of free (unbound) testosterone.

## 3. Effects of Age-Related Decline in Testosterone Levels

The decline in testosterone levels with age can have various effects on the body and overall health. While these effects can vary among individuals, some common manifestations include:

➤ *Sexual Function:*

Reduced testosterone levels can contribute to changes in sexual desire (libido), erectile function, and overall sexual performance. However, it is important to note that other factors, such as chronic health conditions or medications, can also impact sexual function.

➤ *Muscle Mass and Strength:*

Testosterone plays a significant role in maintaining muscle mass and strength. As testosterone levels decline, there is a gradual loss of muscle tissue, leading to decreased muscle strength and potentially an increased risk of sarcopenia (age-related muscle loss).

➤ *Bone Health:*

Testosterone is essential for maintaining healthy bone density. Lower testosterone levels can contribute to a gradual loss of bone mass, potentially leading to osteoporosis and an increased risk of fractures.

➤ *Fat Distribution and Body Composition:*

With declining testosterone levels, there may be an increase in body fat and changes in fat distribution. This can result in a higher proportion of body fat, particularly in the abdominal region, and a decrease in lean muscle mass.

➢ *Mood and Cognitive Function:*

Testosterone has an impact on mood regulation, cognitive function, and overall well-being. Lower testosterone levels have been associated with mood swings, fatigue, irritability, and a higher risk of developing mood disorders such as depression. Some studies have also suggested a potential link between low testosterone levels and cognitive decline.

➢ *Energy Levels and Fatigue:*

Testosterone contributes to overall energy levels and vitality. As testosterone levels decline, individuals may experience a decrease in energy, increased fatigue, and a reduced sense of well-being.

➢ *Metabolic Health:*

Testosterone plays a role in regulating metabolism, including insulin sensitivity and fat metabolism. Lower testosterone levels can contribute to a higher risk of metabolic disorders such as obesity, insulin resistance, and type 2 diabetes.

## 4. Managing Age-Related Testosterone Decline

While the decline in testosterone levels is a natural part of aging, there are strategies that individuals can employ to manage and mitigate the potential effects:

> *Healthy Lifestyle Choices:*

Maintaining a healthy lifestyle can help support optimal testosterone levels. This includes regular exercise, a balanced diet rich in essential nutrients, adequate sleep, stress management, and avoiding excessive alcohol consumption and substance abuse.

> *Resistance and Strength Training:*

Engaging in regular resistance and strength training exercises can help maintain muscle mass, strength, and bone density. Weight-bearing exercises, such as lifting weights, can stimulate testosterone production and support overall musculoskeletal health.

> *Weight Management:*

Maintaining a healthy weight is important for hormonal balance. Excess body fat, especially visceral fat around the abdomen, can contribute to hormonal imbalances, including lower testosterone levels.

> *Regular Physical Activity:*

In addition to resistance training, regular physical activity and cardiovascular exercises can contribute to overall well-being and hormonal balance.

➢ *Stress Reduction:*

Chronic stress can negatively impact testosterone production. Employing stress management techniques such as mindfulness, meditation, and relaxation exercises can help reduce stress levels and support healthy hormone levels.

➢ *Hormone Replacement Therapy (HRT):*

In cases of clinically diagnosed low testosterone levels (hypogonadism) that significantly impact an individual's quality of life, hormone replacement therapy (HRT) may be considered. HRT involves administering testosterone in various forms (e.g., gels, injections) to restore testosterone levels to a more optimal range. This approach should only be pursued under the guidance and supervision of a healthcare professional.

Testosterone levels naturally decline with age, which can have various effects on the body and overall health. Understanding the age-related changes in testosterone levels is crucial for individuals to proactively manage their health and well-being. By adopting a healthy lifestyle, engaging in regular physical activity, and seeking appropriate medical care when needed, individuals can support healthy testosterone levels and mitigate the potential effects of age-related testosterone decline.

## 1.3 The Role of Testosterone in Men's Health and Vitality

Testosterone is a key hormone that plays a fundamental role in men's health and vitality. It is primarily produced in the testes and is responsible for the development and maintenance of various physiological processes in the male body. In this article, we will explore the vital role of testosterone in men's health, including its effects on sexual function, muscle mass, bone density, mood, cognitive function, and overall well-being.

### 1. Sexual Function and Reproduction

One of the primary functions of testosterone is its role in sexual function and reproduction. Testosterone plays a crucial role in:

➢ ***Libido and Sexual Desire:***

Testosterone is responsible for the development of sexual desire (libido) in men. Adequate testosterone levels are essential for a healthy sex drive and overall sexual satisfaction.

➢ ***Erectile Function:***

Testosterone influences erectile function by promoting adequate blood flow to the penis and facilitating the physiological processes required for achieving and maintaining an erection.

 *Sperm Production:*

Testosterone plays a role in the production of sperm cells in the testes. It supports the development and maturation of sperm, which is crucial for fertility and reproduction.

## 2. Muscle Mass and Strength

Testosterone is a key hormone in the regulation of muscle mass and strength. It contributes to:

➤ *Muscle Development:*

Testosterone stimulates protein synthesis, which is essential for muscle growth and development. It promotes the formation of new muscle tissue and helps maintain existing muscle mass.

➤ *Muscle Strength:*

Higher testosterone levels are associated with increased muscle strength and power. Testosterone enhances the activation of muscle fibers, resulting in greater force production and improved athletic performance.

➤ *Prevention of Muscle Wasting:*

Testosterone plays a role in preventing muscle wasting (atrophy). In conditions where testosterone levels are significantly reduced, such as in hypogonadism, there is an increased risk of muscle loss.

## 3. Bone Density and Osteoporosis

Testosterone is crucial for maintaining healthy bone density and preventing the development of osteoporosis, a condition characterized by weakened and brittle bones. Testosterone contributes to:

➤ *Bone Mineralization:*

Testosterone promotes bone mineralization, which involves the deposition of essential minerals like calcium and phosphorus into the bone matrix. This process helps maintain bone strength and integrity.

➤ *Stimulation of Bone Formation:*

Testosterone stimulates the activity of osteoblasts, the cells responsible for bone formation. Adequate testosterone levels are necessary for optimal bone growth and remodeling.

➢ *Prevention of Osteoporosis:*

Low testosterone levels are associated with a higher risk of osteoporosis in men. The gradual decline in testosterone with age contributes to the loss of bone density, making men more susceptible to fractures and bone-related issues.

## 4. Mood, Cognitive Function, and Well-being

Testosterone influences mood, cognitive function, and overall well-being in men. Adequate testosterone levels contribute to:

➢ *Mood Regulation:*

Testosterone plays a role in mood regulation and overall emotional well-being. Optimal testosterone levels are associated with improved mood, increased motivation, and a sense of well-being. Low testosterone levels have been linked to mood disorders, such as depression and irritability.

➢ *Cognitive Function:*

Testosterone influences various cognitive functions, including memory, attention, and spatial abilities. It plays a role in maintaining cognitive health and may contribute to the prevention of cognitive decline and age-related neurodegenerative diseases.

➢ *Energy Levels and Vitality:*

Testosterone is crucial for energy production and overall vitality. Adequate testosterone levels are associated with increased energy, reduced fatigue, and improved overall quality of life.

## 5. Metabolic Health and Body Composition

Testosterone has a significant impact on metabolic health and body composition in men. Influences:

➢ *Fat Distribution:*

Testosterone helps regulate fat distribution in the body. Higher testosterone levels are associated with reduced visceral fat (fat stored around the organs) and a more favorable body composition.

➢ *Insulin Sensitivity:*

Testosterone plays a role in maintaining insulin sensitivity, which is crucial for glucose regulation and preventing the development of insulin resistance and type 2 diabetes.

> ***Metabolic Rate:***

Testosterone influences the metabolic rate, affecting how efficiently the body utilizes energy. Adequate testosterone levels support a healthy metabolic rate, which can contribute to weight management and overall metabolic health.

> ***Lipid Profile:***

Testosterone helps maintain a healthy lipid profile by regulating cholesterol levels. It promotes the production of high-density lipoprotein (HDL) cholesterol, often referred to as "good" cholesterol, while inhibiting the production of low-density lipoprotein (LDL) cholesterol, known as "bad" cholesterol.

## 6. Aging and Testosterone Levels

It is important to note that testosterone levels naturally decline with age. This decline, commonly referred to as andropause or late-onset hypogonadism, can have various effects on men's health and vitality. While the decline is a natural part of aging, some men may experience symptoms related to low testosterone levels. These symptoms may include decreased libido, fatigue, decreased muscle mass and strength, increased body fat, mood changes, and reduced cognitive function.

## 7. Managing Testosterone Levels

Although testosterone levels decline with age, there are strategies that can help support healthy testosterone levels and promote men's health and vitality:

> ***Healthy Lifestyle Choices:***

Adopting a healthy lifestyle is crucial for optimizing testosterone levels. This includes regular exercise, a balanced diet rich in essential nutrients, adequate sleep, stress management, and avoiding excessive alcohol consumption and substance abuse.

> ***Strength Training and Physical Activity:***

Engaging in regular strength training exercises can help maintain muscle mass and strength, supporting healthy testosterone levels. Additionally, regular physical activity, including cardiovascular exercise, can contribute to overall well-being and hormonal balance.

> ***Weight Management:***

Maintaining a healthy weight is important for hormone regulation. Excess body fat, particularly visceral fat, can contribute to hormonal imbalances, including lower testosterone levels.

> ***Stress Reduction:***

Chronic stress can negatively impact testosterone production. Incorporating stress management techniques such as mindfulness, meditation, and relaxation exercises can help reduce stress levels and support healthy hormone levels.

> ***Medical Intervention:***

In cases of clinically diagnosed low testosterone levels (hypogonadism) that significantly impact an individual's quality of life, hormone replacement therapy (HRT) may be considered. HRT involves administering testosterone in various forms (e.g., gels, injections) to restore testosterone levels to a more optimal range. This approach should only be pursued under the guidance and supervision of a healthcare professional.

Testosterone plays a vital role in men's health and vitality, influencing various aspects of sexual function, muscle mass, bone density, mood, cognitive function, metabolic health, and overall well-being. Understanding the importance of testosterone and its effects on men's health is crucial for promoting a healthy and fulfilling life. By adopting a healthy lifestyle, engaging in regular physical activity, and seeking appropriate medical care when needed, men can optimize their testosterone levels and support their health and vitality throughout their lifespan.

# Chapter 2: Factors Affecting Testosterone Levels

Testosterone is a hormone that plays a crucial role in various physiological processes in both males and females. While testosterone levels naturally decline with age, there are several factors that can influence testosterone production and overall levels. In this chapter, we will explore the factors that affect testosterone levels, including lifestyle choices, medical conditions, medications, and environmental factors.

## 1. Lifestyle Factors

> ### ➢ *Diet and Nutrition:*

The type and quality of the diet can impact testosterone levels. Some key factors include:

- Adequate calorie intake: Severely restricted calorie intake can lower testosterone levels, while excessive calorie intake and obesity can lead to imbalances.
- Nutrient intake: Certain nutrients, such as zinc, vitamin D, magnesium, and omega-3 fatty acids, are important for testosterone production. A diet rich in lean proteins, fruits, vegetables, whole grains, and healthy fats can support optimal testosterone levels.
- Avoidance of processed foods: Processed foods, high in refined sugars and unhealthy fats, can contribute to insulin resistance, obesity, and hormonal imbalances, potentially affecting testosterone levels.

➢ *Physical Activity and Exercise:*

Regular physical activity and exercise can have a positive impact on testosterone levels. Factors to consider include:

- Resistance training: Engaging in strength training exercises, such as weightlifting, can stimulate testosterone production and promote muscle growth.
- High-intensity interval training (HIIT): HIIT workouts, involving short bursts of intense exercise, have been shown to increase testosterone levels.
- Overtraining: Excessive exercise and overtraining can lead to hormonal imbalances and decrease testosterone levels. Finding a balance between exercise and recovery is crucial.

➢ *Sleep and Stress Management:*

Quality sleep and stress management play a role in testosterone regulation. Factors to consider include:

- Sufficient sleep: Inadequate sleep and poor sleep quality can disrupt hormonal balance, including testosterone production. Aim for 7-8 hours of uninterrupted sleep each night.
- Stress reduction: Chronic stress can contribute to lower testosterone levels. Employing stress management techniques such as meditation, deep breathing exercises, and engaging in hobbies can help reduce stress levels and support healthy hormone production.

## 2. Medical Conditions and Medications

### ➢ *Hypogonadism:*

Hypogonadism refers to a condition where the body doesn't produce sufficient testosterone. It can be classified as primary (testicular failure) or secondary (hypothalamic-pituitary dysfunction). Causes of hypogonadism include genetic disorders, testicular injury or infection, pituitary or hypothalamic disorders, and certain medical treatments.

### ➢ *Obesity and Metabolic Syndrome:*

Obesity and metabolic syndrome, characterized by central obesity, insulin resistance, high blood pressure, and dyslipidemia, can contribute to lower testosterone levels. Excess body fat, particularly visceral fat, can lead to increased conversion of testosterone to estrogen, resulting in hormonal imbalances.

### ➢ *Chronic Illnesses and Medical Treatments:*

Certain chronic illnesses and medical treatments can impact testosterone levels. These include:

- Diabetes: Poorly controlled diabetes and insulin resistance can affect testosterone production.

- Chronic kidney disease: Kidney disease can disrupt hormonal balance and lower testosterone levels.
- HIV/AIDS: Individuals with HIV/AIDS may experience lower testosterone levels due to the infection itself or as a side effect of antiretroviral therapy.
- Cancer treatments: Chemotherapy, radiation therapy, and hormonal therapies used in the treatment of cancer can lower testosterone levels.

> ***Medications:***

Several medications can affect testosterone levels. Examples include:

- Hormonal medications: Some hormonal medications, such as certain types of birth control pills, can decrease testosterone levels.
- Corticosteroids: Prolonged use of corticosteroids, such as prednisone and dexamethasone, can suppress testosterone production.
- Opioids: Opioid medications, used for pain management, can lower testosterone levels.
- Anti-androgens: Certain medications used in the treatment of prostate cancer or transgender hormone therapy can block the effects of testosterone or decrease testosterone production.

## 3. Environmental Factors

> ***Endocrine Disrupting Chemicals (EDCs):***

Exposure to certain chemicals in the environment, known as endocrine-disrupting chemicals (EDCs), can interfere with hormone production and regulation, including testosterone. EDCs can be found in plastics, pesticides, personal care products, and some food additives. Avoiding or minimizing exposure to these chemicals may help maintain healthy testosterone levels.

> ***Heavy Metals:***

Exposure to heavy metals, such as lead, mercury, and cadmium, can have adverse effects on testosterone production. Occupational exposure or contaminated food and water sources are common routes of exposure. Minimizing exposure to heavy metals is important for overall health and hormonal balance.

> ***Lifestyle Factors:***

Certain lifestyle choices can negatively impact testosterone levels. These include:

- Excessive alcohol consumption: Chronic alcohol abuse can lead to decreased testosterone production and testicular damage.

- Smoking: Cigarette smoking has been associated with lower testosterone levels and hormonal imbalances.
- Substance abuse: Illicit drug use, such as anabolic steroids and opioids, can disrupt testosterone production and hormonal balance.

## 4. Age and Natural Decline

It is important to recognize that testosterone levels naturally decline with age in both males and females. This decline, often referred to as andropause in men, is a normal part of the aging process. While the decline is gradual, it can have various effects on health and well-being. Strategies to manage age-related testosterone decline include lifestyle modifications, regular exercise, and medical interventions if necessary.

Numerous factors can influence testosterone levels in both males and females. Lifestyle factors, such as diet, exercise, sleep, and stress management, play a significant role in maintaining optimal testosterone levels. Additionally, certain medical conditions, medications, and environmental factors can affect testosterone production and regulation. Understanding the factors that influence testosterone levels is essential for promoting hormonal balance and overall health. By making informed choices, seeking appropriate medical care, and minimizing exposure to potential disruptors, individuals can support healthy testosterone levels and optimize their well-being.

## 2.1 Lifestyle and Its Impact on Testosterone

Testosterone is a vital hormone that plays a significant role in various aspects of human health. Lifestyle factors can have a profound impact on testosterone levels. Adopting a healthy lifestyle can support optimal testosterone production and regulation, contributing to overall well-being. In this article, we will explore the influence of lifestyle choices on testosterone levels and provide practical strategies for maintaining healthy testosterone levels through lifestyle modifications.

### 1. Diet and Nutrition

➢ *Adequate Caloric Intake:*

Maintaining an appropriate caloric intake is essential for testosterone production. Severely restricting calories can lead to lower testosterone levels, while excessive calorie consumption can contribute to weight gain and hormonal imbalances. It is important to find a balance and ensure that calorie intake aligns with individual needs.

➢ *Balanced Macronutrient Distribution:*

The distribution of macronutrients in the diet can impact testosterone levels. Key considerations include:

- Protein: Sufficient protein intake is crucial for testosterone production. Include lean meats, poultry, fish, eggs, dairy products, legumes, and plant-based protein sources in the diet.
- Healthy Fats: Adequate intake of healthy fats, such as monounsaturated and polyunsaturated fats found in avocados, nuts, seeds, and fatty fish, is important for hormone production, including testosterone.
- Carbohydrates: Opt for complex carbohydrates, such as whole grains, fruits, and vegetables, which provide essential nutrients and fiber, and help maintain stable blood sugar levels.

> *Micronutrients:*

Certain micronutrients play a role in testosterone production. Include the following in your diet:

- Zinc: Zinc is essential for testosterone synthesis. Good sources include oysters, beef, poultry, beans, nuts, and whole grains.
- Vitamin D: Vitamin D deficiency has been associated with lower testosterone levels. Get adequate sunlight exposure or consider supplementation if necessary.
- Magnesium: Magnesium is involved in testosterone production and regulation. Include magnesium-rich foods such as leafy greens, nuts, seeds, and whole grains in your diet.

> *Limiting Processed Foods and Sugar:*

Processed foods, high in refined sugars and unhealthy fats, can contribute to insulin resistance, obesity, and hormonal imbalances. Limiting the consumption of processed foods and added sugars is crucial for supporting healthy testosterone levels.

## 2. Physical Activity and Exercise

### ➢ *Resistance Training:*

Engaging in regular resistance training exercises, such as weightlifting or bodyweight exercises, can stimulate testosterone production. Resistance training promotes muscle growth and strength, which is associated with higher testosterone levels.

### ➢ *High-Intensity Interval Training (HIIT):*

HIIT workouts involve short bursts of intense exercise followed by brief recovery periods. Incorporating HIIT exercises into your fitness routine can increase testosterone levels more effectively compared to steady-state cardio exercises.

### ➢ *Moderate Aerobic Exercise:*

While resistance training and HIIT are beneficial, moderate aerobic exercises like jogging, swimming, or cycling can also support overall health and hormonal balance. Aim for a combination of resistance training, HIIT, and aerobic exercises to maximize the benefits for testosterone levels.

> ### *Avoid Overtraining:*

Excessive exercise and overtraining can lead to hormonal imbalances and lower testosterone levels. It is important to find the right balance between exercise and recovery. Allow adequate rest days and listen to your body's signals.

## 3. Sleep and Stress Management

> ### *Sufficient Sleep:*

Quality sleep is crucial for hormonal balance, including testosterone production. Aim for 7-8 hours of uninterrupted sleep each night. Create a sleep-friendly environment, establish a consistent sleep schedule, and practice good sleep hygiene to promote restful sleep.

> ### *Stress Reduction*:

Chronic stress can disrupt hormone production and lead to lower testosterone levels. Implement stress reduction techniques such as meditation, deep breathing exercises, yoga, or engaging in hobbies and activities that promote relaxation. Find healthy outlets to manage stress and prioritize self-care.

> *Work-Life Balance:*

Maintaining a healthy work-life balance is essential for managing stress levels. Find ways to prioritize personal time, hobbies, and relationships outside of work to reduce chronic stress and support hormonal balance.

> *Mindfulness and Relaxation:*

Incorporate mindfulness practices and relaxation techniques into your daily routine. This can include mindfulness meditation, progressive muscle relaxation, or engaging in activities that promote relaxation and mental well-being.

## 4. Weight Management

> *Achieving and Maintaining a Healthy Weight:*

Excess body weight, especially visceral fat, can contribute to hormonal imbalances, including lower testosterone levels. Aim to achieve and maintain a healthy weight through a combination of a balanced diet and regular exercise.

> *Focus on Body Composition:*

Focus on body composition rather than just weight loss. Prioritize building and maintaining lean muscle mass through resistance training, which can support testosterone production and metabolic health.

## 5. Limiting Alcohol and Substance Use

> ➢ *Alcohol Consumption:*

Excessive alcohol consumption can negatively impact testosterone levels. Limit alcohol intake or practice moderation to support healthy testosterone production. Guidelines suggest that men should limit alcohol consumption to no more than two drinks per day.

> ➢ *Substance Abuse:*

Illicit drug use, including anabolic steroids and opioids, can disrupt testosterone production and hormonal balance. Avoid substance abuse and seek help if you are struggling with addiction.

## 6. Smoking Cessation

Cigarette smoking has been associated with lower testosterone levels. Quitting smoking can improve overall health and support hormonal balance, including testosterone production. Seek support from healthcare professionals or smoking cessation programs to quit smoking.

Lifestyle choices have a significant impact on testosterone levels. Adopting a healthy lifestyle that includes a balanced diet, regular physical activity, sufficient sleep, stress management, and avoiding excessive alcohol and substance use can support optimal testosterone production and regulation. By making informed choices and prioritizing self-care, individuals can maintain healthy testosterone levels, promoting overall health, vitality, and well-being.

**2.2 Nutrition and Testosterone-Boosting Foods**

Proper nutrition plays a crucial role in maintaining optimal testosterone levels. Certain nutrients and foods have been found to support testosterone production and regulation in the body. In this article, we will explore the impact of nutrition on testosterone levels and provide a comprehensive list of testosterone-boosting foods that can be incorporated into a healthy diet.

**1. Key Nutrients for Testosterone Production**

➢ *Zinc:*

Zinc is a vital mineral that supports testosterone production. It plays a role in the synthesis of luteinizing hormone (LH), which stimulates testosterone production in the testes. Foods rich in zinc include oysters, beef, poultry, seafood (such as crab and lobster), pumpkin seeds, nuts (such as almonds and cashews), and legumes (such as chickpeas and lentils).

➢ *Vitamin D:*

Vitamin D is important for overall health and has been linked to testosterone production. Foods naturally rich in vitamin D include fatty fish (such as salmon, mackerel, and sardines), egg yolks, and fortified dairy products. Additionally, getting adequate sunlight exposure can help the body produce vitamin D.

➢ *Magnesium:*

Magnesium is involved in numerous physiological processes, including testosterone production. It supports the conversion of cholesterol into testosterone in the testes. Magnesium-rich foods include leafy greens (such as spinach and kale), nuts (such as almonds and cashews), seeds (such as pumpkin seeds and flaxseeds), whole grains, and legumes.

➢ *Vitamin K2:*

Vitamin K2 has been associated with increased testosterone levels. It can be found in fermented foods like natto, cheese, and sauerkraut. Additionally, certain animal products, such as grass-fed butter and organ meats, are good sources of vitamin K2.

## 2. Testosterone-Boosting Foods

### ➢ *Lean Meats and Poultry:*

Lean meats, such as beef, chicken, and turkey, are excellent sources of protein, zinc, and vitamin B12, all of which support testosterone production. Choose lean cuts of meat and poultry to reduce saturated fat intake.

### ➢ *Fatty Fish:*

Fatty fish, including salmon, mackerel, and sardines, are rich in omega-3 fatty acids, which have been associated with increased testosterone levels. These fish also provide vitamin D and protein, further supporting testosterone production.

### ➢ *Eggs:*

Eggs are a nutrient-dense food that contains protein, healthy fats, vitamin D, and vitamin B5, all of which can contribute to testosterone production. Opt for whole eggs, as the yolk contains most of the nutrients.

### ➢ *Shellfish:*

Shellfish, such as oysters, crabs, and lobsters, are known for their high zinc content. Zinc is essential for testosterone synthesis and maintaining healthy sperm levels. Including shellfish in the diet can support testosterone production.

> **Nuts and Seeds:**

Nuts and seeds, such as almonds, walnuts, pumpkin seeds, and flaxseeds, provide a combination of healthy fats, protein, and essential minerals like zinc and magnesium. Snacking on these nutritious options can positively impact testosterone levels.

> *Cruciferous Vegetables:*

Cruciferous vegetables, including broccoli, cauliflower, cabbage, and Brussels sprouts, contain compounds that may help regulate estrogen levels. By promoting a healthy estrogen balance, these vegetables indirectly support testosterone production.

> *Legumes:*

Legumes, such as chickpeas, lentils, and beans, are high in protein and fiber. They also provide zinc and magnesium, which are important for testosterone production. Including legumes in the diet can contribute to overall hormonal balance.

➢ *Leafy Greens:*

Leafy greens, such as spinach, kale, and Swiss chard, are rich in magnesium, vitamin K, and other nutrients that support testosterone production. These greens are also low in calories and high in fiber, making them a nutritious addition to any diet.

➢ *Avocados:*

Avocados are a great source of healthy fats, including monounsaturated fats, which support testosterone production. They also provide essential nutrients like vitamin K, vitamin E, and potassium.

➢ *Berries:*

Berries, such as strawberries, blueberries, and raspberries, are packed with antioxidants that help reduce inflammation and support overall health. They also contain fiber and other nutrients that can positively impact testosterone levels indirectly.

➢ *Garlic:*

Garlic has been shown to have potential testosterone-boosting properties. It contains compounds that may help stimulate testosterone production and improve sperm quality. Incorporate garlic into your cooking or consider garlic supplements.

➢ *Pomegranates:*

Pomegranates are rich in antioxidants and can have a positive impact on testosterone levels. Studies have suggested that pomegranate juice may increase testosterone levels and improve overall sexual health.

➢ *Dark Chocolate:*

Dark chocolate, with a high percentage of cocoa, contains flavonoids that have been linked to increased testosterone levels. Additionally, dark chocolate is rich in antioxidants and can provide other health benefits when consumed in moderation.

➢ *Olive Oil:*

Olive oil is a healthy source of monounsaturated fats, which support testosterone production. Use olive oil as a cooking oil or drizzle it over salads and vegetables for added flavor and nutritional benefits.

## 3. Dietary Considerations

➢ *Balanced Diet:*

Maintaining a balanced diet that includes a variety of whole foods is crucial for overall health and hormone production. Incorporate testosterone-boosting foods while ensuring a well-rounded and nutrient-dense diet.

> ***Caloric Intake:***

Maintain a healthy and appropriate caloric intake to support testosterone production. Severely restricting calories can negatively impact hormone production, while excessive calorie intake can lead to weight gain and hormonal imbalances.

> **Nutrient Timing:**

Consider nutrient timing, particularly around exercise. Consuming a combination of protein and carbohydrates before and after workouts can support muscle growth and testosterone production.

> ***Hydration:***

Stay hydrated to support overall health and hormonal balance. Aim to drink an adequate amount of water throughout the day.

> ***Limit Processed Foods and Added Sugars:***

Processed foods and added sugars can contribute to weight gain, insulin resistance, and hormonal imbalances. Minimize the consumption of processed foods and opt for whole, unprocessed options whenever possible.

Proper nutrition plays a significant role in maintaining optimal testosterone levels. Including testosterone-boosting foods, such as lean meats, fatty fish, eggs, nuts, seeds, cruciferous vegetables, and pomegranates, in a balanced diet can support testosterone production and overall health. It is important to prioritize nutrient-dense whole foods, maintain a healthy caloric intake, and make lifestyle choices that support hormonal balance. Consulting with a healthcare professional or registered dietitian can provide personalized guidance for optimizing nutrition and supporting testosterone levels.

## 2.3 Exercise and Its Effect on Testosterone Production

Regular exercise is known to have numerous health benefits, including its impact on hormone regulation. Specifically, exercise has been shown to influence testosterone production in both men and women. In this article, we will explore the relationship between exercise and testosterone production, the types of exercise that are most effective, and how to optimize exercise routines for maximizing testosterone levels.

## 1. Understanding Testosterone

Testosterone is a hormone primarily produced in the testes in men and in the ovaries and adrenal glands in women. It plays a crucial role in the development and maintenance of secondary sexual characteristics, as well as the regulation of various physiological processes. Testosterone is involved in muscle development, bone density, sexual function, mood regulation, and overall well-being.

## 2. How Exercise Affects Testosterone Production

### ➢ *Resistance Training:*

Resistance training, such as weightlifting or bodyweight exercises, has been shown to have a positive impact on testosterone levels. Key effects of resistance training include:

- Increased testosterone production: Intense resistance training stimulates the release of testosterone, leading to a temporary increase in testosterone levels post-workout.
- Muscle development: Resistance training promotes muscle growth, and increased muscle mass is associated with higher testosterone levels.
- Metabolic benefits: Resistance training can improve insulin sensitivity and metabolic health, which can positively impact testosterone production.

### ➢ *High-Intensity Interval Training (HIIT):*

HIIT workouts involve short bursts of intense exercise followed by brief recovery periods. HIIT has been found to stimulate testosterone production and provide metabolic benefits. The effects of HIIT on testosterone include:

- Increased testosterone production: HIIT workouts can trigger a hormonal response that leads to increased testosterone levels.

- Enhanced fat loss: HIIT has been associated with improvements in body composition, including reductions in body fat, which can indirectly support testosterone levels.
- Metabolic benefits: HIIT workouts can improve insulin sensitivity and cardiovascular health, which can positively impact testosterone production.

> ***Endurance Training:***

Endurance exercises, such as running, cycling, or swimming, can also influence testosterone levels. However, the effects of endurance training on testosterone production are different from those of resistance training and HIIT:

- Moderate-intensity endurance training: Moderate-intensity endurance exercises have been found to have a positive impact on testosterone levels, particularly in untrained individuals. The effects are less pronounced compared to resistance training and HIIT.
- Prolonged and intense endurance training: Intense and prolonged endurance training, such as marathon running or high-volume training, can temporarily suppress testosterone production. This is often referred to as the "overtraining syndrome" and may lead to hormonal imbalances.

### 3. Optimizing Exercise Routines for Testosterone Production

➢ **Resistance Training:**

To maximize the testosterone-boosting effects of resistance training:

- Focus on compound exercises: Compound exercises, such as squats, deadlifts, bench presses, and pull-ups, engage multiple muscle groups and stimulate testosterone production more effectively than isolated exercises.
- Lift heavy weights: Lift weights that challenge your muscles and allow for 6-12 repetitions per set. Using heavier weights with proper form can promote greater testosterone release.
- Include full-body workouts: Incorporate exercises that target different muscle groups in a single workout session to stimulate testosterone production throughout the body.
- Allow for adequate recovery: Give your muscles time to rest and recover between resistance training sessions. Overtraining can lead to reduced testosterone production.

➢ **HIIT:**

To optimize HIIT workouts for testosterone production:

- Perform short, intense intervals: Focus on short bursts of high-intensity exercise followed by brief recovery periods. This pattern has been shown to elicit a favorable hormonal response.

- Vary exercises and intensity: Incorporate a mix of exercises and intensities to keep your body challenged and stimulate testosterone production. This can include exercises like sprints, burpees, kettlebell swings, or jumping jacks.
- Limit frequency: HIIT workouts can be demanding on the body, so it is important to allow for proper recovery between sessions. Aim for 2-3 HIIT workouts per week.

## ➢ *Endurance Training:*

To balance the effects of endurance training on testosterone production:

- Include resistance training: Incorporate regular resistance training sessions alongside your endurance workouts to maintain muscle mass and support testosterone levels.
- Moderate intensity: Aim for moderate-intensity endurance training rather than prolonged, high-intensity sessions to minimize the risk of hormonal imbalances.
- Monitor training volume: Be mindful of the volume and intensity of your endurance training. Avoid excessive training loads and allow for adequate rest and recovery.

## 4. Other Factors to Consider

## ➢ *Nutrition:*

Supporting testosterone production through proper nutrition is crucial. Ensure a balanced diet that includes adequate protein, healthy fats, and essential vitamins and minerals like zinc, vitamin D, and magnesium. Refer to the "Nutrition and Testosterone-Boosting Foods" section for more details.

> ### *Sleep and Stress Management:*

Prioritize quality sleep and manage stress effectively. Poor sleep and chronic stress can disrupt hormone regulation, including testosterone production. Aim for 7-8 hours of uninterrupted sleep each night and incorporate stress reduction techniques such as meditation, deep breathing exercises, or engaging in hobbies and activities that promote relaxation.

> ### *Lifestyle Factors:*

Maintain a healthy lifestyle by limiting alcohol consumption, avoiding smoking, and minimizing exposure to environmental factors that can disrupt hormone balance. These factors can have a negative impact on testosterone production and overall health.

> ### *Consistency and Progression:*

Consistency is key to maintaining optimal testosterone levels. Stick to a regular exercise routine and gradually progress in terms of intensity and volume. Consistent exercise over time is more effective for boosting testosterone levels than sporadic or infrequent workouts.

Exercise has a significant impact on testosterone production, and different types of exercise can influence testosterone levels in unique ways. Resistance training and HIIT workouts have been shown to be particularly effective for stimulating testosterone production, while moderate-intensity endurance training can also have positive effects. By incorporating a balanced exercise routine, optimizing workouts for testosterone production, and considering other lifestyle factors, individuals can support healthy testosterone levels and promote overall well-being. It is important to consult with a healthcare professional or a qualified fitness trainer to tailor exercise routines based on individual needs and goals.

# Chapter 3: Natural Methods for Boosting Testosterone

Maintaining healthy testosterone levels is important for both men and women. While medical interventions such as hormone replacement therapy exist, there are also natural methods that can support testosterone production. In this chapter, we will explore various natural methods for boosting testosterone, including lifestyle changes, dietary modifications, supplementation, stress management techniques, and sleep optimization.

## 1. Lifestyle Changes

➢ *Regular Exercise:*

Engaging in regular physical activity, including resistance training and high-intensity interval training (HIIT), can stimulate testosterone production. Aim for at least 150 minutes of moderate-intensity aerobic exercise or 75 minutes of vigorous-intensity exercise per week, along with two or more days of strength training.

> ➢ *Weight Management:*

Maintaining a healthy weight is important for testosterone regulation. Excess body fat, especially visceral fat, can contribute to hormonal imbalances. Focus on a balanced diet and regular exercise to achieve and maintain a healthy weight.

> ➢ *Stress Reduction:*

Chronic stress can negatively impact testosterone levels. Incorporate stress management techniques such as mindfulness meditation, deep breathing exercises, yoga, or engaging in hobbies and activities that promote relaxation. Find healthy outlets to manage stress and prioritize self-care.

> ➢ *Adequate Sleep:*

Quality sleep is crucial for hormone regulation, including testosterone production. Aim for 7-8 hours of uninterrupted sleep each night. Create a sleep-friendly environment, establish a consistent sleep schedule, and practice good sleep hygiene to promote restful sleep.

➢ *Limit Alcohol Consumption:*

Excessive alcohol consumption can have a negative impact on testosterone levels. Practice moderation and limit alcohol intake to support healthy testosterone production. Guidelines suggest that men should limit alcohol consumption to no more than two drinks per day.

## 2. Dietary Modifications

➢ *Balanced Diet:*

Follow a balanced diet that includes a variety of nutrient-dense foods. Focus on whole foods such as fruits, vegetables, lean proteins, whole grains, and healthy fats. A well-rounded diet can support overall health and hormone production.

➢ *Testosterone-Boosting Foods:*

Incorporate foods that are known to support testosterone production. Examples include lean meats, fatty fish (rich in omega-3 fatty acids), eggs, shellfish (rich in zinc), nuts and seeds (rich in healthy fats and minerals), cruciferous vegetables, avocados, and berries (rich in antioxidants). Refer to the "Nutrition and Testosterone-Boosting Foods" section for more details.

➤ *Adequate Nutrient Intake:*

Ensure sufficient intake of key nutrients involved in testosterone production, such as zinc, vitamin D, magnesium, and vitamin K2. Consider supplementation if necessary, but consult with a healthcare professional to determine the appropriate dosage and duration.

➤ *Avoid Excessive Caloric Restriction:*

Severely restricting calorie intake can lead to lower testosterone levels. It is important to maintain an appropriate caloric intake that supports overall health and hormone production. Consult with a registered dietitian for personalized guidance.

## 3. Stress Management Techniques

➤ *Mindfulness Meditation:*

Practicing mindfulness meditation can help reduce stress levels and promote overall well-being. Set aside time each day for meditation, focusing on the present moment and observing thoughts and sensations without judgment.

➤ *Deep Breathing Exercises:*

Deep breathing exercises, such as diaphragmatic breathing or box breathing, can activate the body's relaxation response and help reduce stress. Incorporate these exercises into your daily routine or during moments of stress.

> ***Yoga and Tai Chi:***

Yoga and Tai Chi combine physical movement, breath control, and mindfulness, offering a holistic approach to stress management. Regular practice can help reduce stress and promote a sense of calm.

> ***Engaging in Hobbies and Relaxation Activities:***

Participating in activities that bring joy and relaxation can help alleviate stress and promote a positive mood. Find activities that you enjoy, such as listening to music, painting, gardening, or spending time in nature, and make time for them regularly.

## 4. Sleep Optimization

> ***Establish a Consistent Sleep Schedule:***

Maintain a regular sleep routine by going to bed and waking up at the same time every day, even on weekends. This helps regulate the body's internal clock and promotes better sleep quality.

➢ *Create a Sleep-Friendly Environment:*

Ensure your bedroom is dark, quiet, and cool. Use blackout curtains, earplugs, or white noise machines if necessary. Remove electronic devices that emit blue light, as this can interfere with sleep.

➢ *Practice Relaxation Techniques Before Bed:*

Engage in activities that promote relaxation before bedtime. This can include reading a book, taking a warm bath, practicing relaxation exercises, or listening to calming music. Avoid stimulating activities or bright screens close to bedtime.

➢ *Limit Caffeine and Stimulants:*

Avoid consuming caffeine or other stimulants close to bedtime, as they can interfere with sleep. Opt for herbal teas or other caffeine-free alternatives in the evening.

## 5. Considerations for Supplementation

➢ *Consult with a Healthcare Professional:*

Before considering any supplementation, it is important to consult with a healthcare professional. They can assess your individual needs, review your medical history, and determine if supplementation is necessary or appropriate.

> ### ➢ *Vitamin D:*

If you have low vitamin D levels, supplementation may be recommended. However, it is best to have your vitamin D levels tested and work with a healthcare professional to determine the appropriate dosage.

> ### ➢ *Zinc and Magnesium:*

Zinc and magnesium are minerals involved in testosterone production. If you have deficiencies or inadequate intake of these minerals, supplementation may be considered. Work with a healthcare professional to determine the appropriate dosage.

> ### ➢ *D-Aspartic Acid:*

D-Aspartic acid is an amino acid that has been shown to support testosterone production in some studies. However, more research is needed to establish its effectiveness and safety. Consult with a healthcare professional before considering supplementation.

Boosting testosterone levels naturally involves making lifestyle changes, modifying dietary habits, managing stress effectively, optimizing sleep, and considering supplementation when appropriate. By incorporating these natural methods, individuals can support healthy testosterone production and promote overall well-being. It is important to consult with healthcare professionals, such as registered dietitians or doctors, for personalized guidance and to ensure safety and efficacy. Remember that results may vary, and consistency is key to maintaining long-term benefits.

## 3.1 Sleep and Its Influence on Testosterone

Sleep is a fundamental aspect of our daily lives and plays a crucial role in maintaining overall health and well-being. In addition to its impact on physical and mental health, sleep also influences hormone regulation, including testosterone production. In this article, we will explore the relationship between sleep and testosterone, the effects of sleep deprivation on testosterone levels, and strategies for optimizing sleep to support healthy testosterone production.

## 1. Understanding Testosterone

Testosterone is a hormone primarily produced in the testes in men and in the ovaries and adrenal glands in women. It is involved in numerous physiological processes, including the development and maintenance of secondary sexual characteristics, muscle growth, bone density, mood regulation, and overall well-being. Testosterone levels naturally fluctuate throughout the day and are influenced by various factors, including sleep.

## 2. The Sleep-Testosterone Connection

➤ *Testosterone Production during Sleep:*

Testosterone production follows a circadian rhythm, with the highest levels typically occurring in the early morning hours, during deep sleep stages. During sleep, the body undergoes important restorative processes, including hormone regulation and tissue repair. Disruptions in sleep can impact testosterone production.

➤ *The Role of Sleep in Hormone Regulation:*

Sleep is vital for proper hormone regulation, including testosterone production. Sleep deprivation or poor sleep quality can disrupt the delicate balance of hormones in the body, leading to hormonal imbalances and potentially affecting testosterone levels.

➤ *Sleep Architecture and Testosterone:*

Sleep is characterized by different stages, including rapid eye movement (REM) sleep and non-rapid eye movement (NREM) sleep. Deep NREM sleep, also known as slow-wave sleep (SWS), is particularly important for hormone regulation and testosterone production. Disruptions in sleep architecture, such as reduced SWS, can influence testosterone levels.

## 3. Effects of Sleep Deprivation on Testosterone

> ***Reduced Testosterone Production:***

Sleep deprivation has been linked to decreased testosterone levels. Several studies have shown that both acute and chronic sleep deprivation can lead to lower testosterone levels in men. Sleep restriction can disrupt the normal sleep-testosterone relationship and negatively impact testosterone production.

> ***Altered Hormone Regulation:***

Sleep deprivation can disrupt the balance of other hormones involved in testosterone regulation, such as luteinizing hormone (LH) and follicle-stimulating hormone (FSH). Decreased LH levels have been observed in individuals experiencing sleep loss, which can subsequently impact testosterone production.

> ***Metabolic Effects:***

Sleep deprivation can also lead to metabolic disturbances, such as insulin resistance and increased cortisol levels. These metabolic changes can further contribute to hormonal imbalances and potentially affect testosterone production.

## 4. Optimizing Sleep for Healthy Testosterone Levels

> ➤ *Prioritize Sufficient Sleep Duration:*

Ensure that you are getting enough sleep on a regular basis. Aim for 7-8 hours of uninterrupted sleep each night, as this is the recommended duration for most adults. However, individual sleep needs may vary, so listen to your body's signals and adjust accordingly.

> ➤ *Establish a Consistent Sleep Schedule:*

Maintain a regular sleep routine by going to bed and waking up at the same time each day, even on weekends. This helps regulate the body's internal clock and promotes better sleep quality.

> ➤ *Create a Sleep-Friendly Environment:*

Ensure that your bedroom is conducive to sleep. Create a cool, dark, and quiet environment that promotes relaxation. Use blackout curtains, earplugs, or white noise machines if necessary. Remove electronic devices that emit blue light, as this can interfere with sleep.

> ➤ *Practice Relaxation Techniques Before Bed:*

Engage in activities that promote relaxation and signal to your body that it's time to sleep. This can include reading a book, taking a warm bath, practicing relaxation exercises such as deep breathing or progressive muscle relaxation, or listening to calming music. Avoid stimulating activities or bright screens close to bedtime.

> *Limit Stimulants and Optimize Nutrition:*

Avoid consuming stimulants such as caffeine or nicotine close to bedtime, as they can interfere with sleep quality. Additionally, be mindful of your diet and nutrition throughout the day, as certain nutrients and foods can support healthy sleep patterns.

> *Manage Stress and Establish a Bedtime Routine:*

Implement stress management techniques such as mindfulness meditation, journaling, or engaging in relaxing activities before bed. Establishing a consistent bedtime routine can signal to your body that it's time to wind down and prepare for sleep.

> *Regular Exercise:*

Engaging in regular physical activity can promote better sleep quality and support testosterone production. Aim for at least 150 minutes of moderate-intensity aerobic exercise or 75 minutes of vigorous-intensity exercise per week. However, avoid exercising too close to bedtime, as it can be stimulating and interfere with sleep.

➢ *Limit Alcohol and Fluid Intake:*

While alcohol may initially make you feel drowsy, it can disrupt sleep patterns and lead to fragmented and less restorative sleep. Limit alcohol consumption, particularly close to bedtime. Additionally, manage fluid intake to minimize nighttime awakenings due to excessive urination.

➢ *Consider Sleep Disorders and Seek Medical Evaluation:*

If you suspect you have a sleep disorder, such as sleep apnea or insomnia, it is important to seek medical evaluation and treatment. Sleep disorders can significantly impact sleep quality and hormone regulation, including testosterone production.

Sleep plays a vital role in testosterone regulation and overall health. Insufficient sleep duration or poor sleep quality can disrupt hormone balance and negatively impact testosterone levels. By prioritizing sufficient sleep, establishing a consistent sleep routine, creating a sleep-friendly environment, practicing relaxation techniques, managing stress, and optimizing nutrition and exercise, individuals can support healthy sleep patterns and promote optimal testosterone production. It is important to prioritize sleep as an integral part of a comprehensive approach to overall well-being.

**3.2 Stress Management Techniques for Optimizing Testosterone**

Chronic stress can have detrimental effects on overall health and well-being, including hormone regulation. Stress can disrupt the delicate balance of hormones in the body, leading to hormonal imbalances, including reduced testosterone levels. In this article, we will explore stress management techniques that can help optimize testosterone levels and promote overall health and vitality.

### 1. Understanding Stress and Testosterone

> *The Impact of Chronic Stress on Testosterone:*

Chronic stress, whether physical or psychological, can lead to dysregulation of the hypothalamic-pituitary-adrenal (HPA) axis, which plays a crucial role in hormone regulation. Stress triggers the release of cortisol, a hormone that helps the body cope with stress. However, prolonged elevation of cortisol levels can interfere with testosterone production, leading to decreased testosterone levels.

> *The Importance of Testosterone Regulation:*

Testosterone is a hormone that plays a vital role in various aspects of health, including muscle growth, bone density, sexual function, mood regulation, and overall well-being. Optimizing testosterone levels is important for both men and women to support overall health and vitality.

## 2. Stress Management Techniques

### ➢ *Mindfulness Meditation:*

Mindfulness meditation involves focusing on the present moment without judgment. It has been shown to reduce stress levels and promote overall well-being. By practicing mindfulness meditation regularly, individuals can learn to manage stress more effectively and promote hormone balance, including testosterone production.

### ➢ *Deep Breathing Exercises:*

Deep breathing exercises, such as diaphragmatic breathing or box breathing, can activate the body's relaxation response and help reduce stress. By taking slow, deep breaths and focusing on the breath, individuals can promote a sense of calm and reduce the impact of stress on hormone regulation.

### ➢ *Progressive Muscle Relaxation (PMR):*

PMR is a technique that involves tensing and then relaxing different muscle groups in the body, promoting physical and mental relaxation. By systematically relaxing the muscles, individuals can release tension and reduce stress levels, supporting overall hormone balance.

> *Yoga and Tai Chi:*

Yoga and Tai Chi combine physical movement, breath control, and mindfulness, offering a holistic approach to stress management. These practices can help reduce stress, promote relaxation, and support hormone regulation, including testosterone production.

> *Exercise and Physical Activity:*

Engaging in regular exercise and physical activity can help reduce stress levels and optimize testosterone production. Exercise promotes the release of endorphins, which are natural mood enhancers. It can also provide a distraction from daily stressors and promote a sense of well-being.

> *Social Support and Connection:*

Maintaining social connections and seeking support from friends, family, or support groups can help reduce stress levels. Sharing feelings and experiences with others can provide emotional support and help manage stress more effectively.

> *Time Management and Prioritization:*

Effective time management and prioritization can help reduce stress levels by creating a sense of control and organization. Breaking tasks into manageable chunks, setting realistic goals, and practicing effective time management techniques can help reduce stress and promote hormonal balance.


> ### *Healthy Lifestyle Habits:*

Adopting healthy lifestyle habits can support stress management and optimize testosterone levels. This includes maintaining a balanced diet, getting regular exercise, practicing good sleep hygiene, limiting alcohol and caffeine consumption, and avoiding smoking or substance abuse.


## 3. Seeking Professional Help


> ### *Counseling and Therapy:*

In some cases, chronic stress and its impact on testosterone levels may require professional intervention. Seeking counseling or therapy can provide individuals with tools and strategies to manage stress effectively and promote hormonal balance.


> ### *Medical Evaluation and Treatment:*

If chronic stress persists or is severe, it is important to seek medical evaluation. A healthcare professional can assess overall health, evaluate hormonal balance, and determine if additional medical interventions are necessary, such as medication or hormone therapy, to address the effects of stress on testosterone levels.

Stress management techniques play a crucial role in optimizing testosterone levels and promoting overall health and vitality. Chronic stress can disrupt hormone regulation, including testosterone production, leading to various health issues. By incorporating stress management techniques such as mindfulness meditation, deep breathing exercises, and progressive muscle relaxation, yoga, and regular physical activity, individuals can effectively manage stress and support hormone balance. Additionally, maintaining a healthy lifestyle, seeking social support, practicing effective time management, and considering professional help when necessary can further enhance stress management and promote optimal testosterone levels. It is important to prioritize stress management as an integral part of overall well-being and make it a regular practice in daily life.

## 3.3 Herbal Supplements and Their Testosterone-Enhancing Properties

Herbal supplements have been used for centuries in traditional medicine systems to promote various aspects of health, including hormone regulation. When it comes to testosterone enhancement, several herbal supplements have gained attention for their potential to support healthy testosterone levels. In this article, we will explore some popular herbal supplements known for their testosterone-enhancing properties, their mechanisms of action, potential benefits, and considerations for use.

### 1. Tribulus Terrestris

Tribulus Terrestris, also known as puncture vine, is a plant native to certain regions of Asia, Europe, and Africa. It has long been used in traditional medicine for its potential to enhance sexual health and improve athletic performance. Tribulus Terrestris is believed to influence testosterone levels through the following mechanisms:

> *Stimulation of Luteinizing Hormone (LH) Production:*

Tribulus Terrestris may stimulate the production of luteinizing hormone (LH) in the body. LH plays a key role in testosterone production, as it signals the testes to produce testosterone.

> *Increased Nitric Oxide (NO) Production:*

Tribulus Terrestris may enhance the release of nitric oxide (NO), which can support blood flow and oxygenation. Improved blood flow can promote overall health and potentially enhance sexual function and performance.

While some studies have shown positive effects of Tribulus terrestris on testosterone levels, other studies have reported conflicting results. More research is needed to establish its effectiveness and determine the appropriate dosage and duration of use.

## 2. Ashwagandha

Ashwagandha, scientifically known as Withania somnifera, is an herb widely used in Ayurvedic medicine. It is revered for its adaptogenic properties, which help the body adapt to stress and promote overall well-being. Ashwagandha may also influence testosterone levels through various mechanisms:

> *Stress Reduction:*

Ashwagandha has been shown to help reduce stress and cortisol levels. Chronic stress and elevated cortisol can negatively impact testosterone production. By reducing stress, ashwagandha may indirectly support healthy testosterone levels.

> *Antioxidant Effects:*

Ashwagandha has antioxidant properties, which can help protect the body from oxidative damage. Oxidative stress can contribute to hormonal imbalances, including decreased testosterone levels. The antioxidant effects of ashwagandha may help maintain optimal testosterone levels.

Several studies have shown promising results in terms of ashwagandha's impact on testosterone levels and reproductive health. However, more research is needed to confirm these findings and determine the optimal dosage and duration of use.

## 3. Fenugreek

Fenugreek (Trigonella foenum-graecum) is an herb commonly used in Indian and Mediterranean cuisine. It has also been used in traditional medicine systems to support male health and vitality. Fenugreek may influence testosterone levels through the following mechanisms:

> ***Stimulation of Testosterone Production:***

Fenugreek contains compounds that can stimulate testosterone production. It is believed to work by blocking the enzyme aromatase, which converts testosterone into estrogen. By inhibiting aromatase activity, fenugreek may help maintain higher testosterone levels.

> ***Regulation of Blood Sugar Levels:***

Fenugreek has been shown to help regulate blood sugar levels. High blood sugar levels can negatively impact testosterone production. By supporting healthy blood sugar regulation, fenugreek may indirectly promote optimal testosterone levels.

Studies investigating fenugreek's effects on testosterone have shown mixed results. While some studies have reported increases in testosterone levels, others have found no significant changes. Further research is needed to better understand fenugreek's potential benefits and establish appropriate dosage guidelines.

## 4. Tongkat Ali

Tongkat Ali, scientifically known as Eurycoma longifolia, is a herb native to Southeast Asia. It has been traditionally used as an aphrodisiac and to enhance male sexual health. Tongkat Ali may impact testosterone levels through the following mechanisms:

> ***Stimulation of Testosterone Production:***

Tongkat Ali contains compounds that can stimulate the release of luteinizing hormone (LH), which in turn promotes testosterone production. By increasing LH levels, Tongkat Ali may support healthy testosterone levels.

> ***Anti-Estrogenic Effects:***

Tongkat Ali may have anti-estrogenic properties, meaning it can help reduce estrogen levels. Estrogen is a hormone that can compete with testosterone, and high estrogen levels can lead to hormonal imbalances. By modulating estrogen levels, Tongkat Ali may help maintain a favorable testosterone-to-estrogen ratio.

Research on Tongkat Ali's effects on testosterone has shown promising results. Studies have reported increases in testosterone levels, improvements in sexual function, and enhanced muscle strength. However, more research is needed to establish optimal dosages and long-term safety.

## 5. Considerations and Precautions

> ***Quality and Dosage:***

When using herbal supplements, it is important to choose high-quality products from reputable sources. Look for standardized extracts and follow the recommended dosage instructions. Consulting with a healthcare professional or herbalist can provide personalized guidance.

➤ *Individual Variations:*

Each individual may respond differently to herbal supplements. Factors such as overall health, age, and underlying hormonal imbalances can influence the effectiveness of these supplements. It is important to monitor how your body responds and adjust accordingly.

➤ *Potential Side Effects:*

While herbal supplements are generally considered safe, they may still have potential side effects. Common side effects can include gastrointestinal discomfort, allergic reactions, or interactions with medications. It is important to be aware of any potential interactions or contraindications, especially if you have underlying health conditions or are taking medications.

➤ *Complementary Approach:*

Herbal supplements should be viewed as part of a comprehensive approach to overall health. It is essential to prioritize a healthy lifestyle, including a balanced diet, regular exercise, stress management, and sufficient sleep. These lifestyle factors can have a significant impact on hormone regulation, including testosterone production.

Herbal supplements such as Tribulus Terrestris, Ashwagandha, Fenugreek, and Tongkat Ali have gained popularity for their potential testosterone-enhancing properties. While they may offer benefits in supporting healthy testosterone levels, it is important to approach their use with caution and under the guidance of a healthcare professional. Herbal supplements should be viewed as part of a holistic approach to overall health, including lifestyle modifications and stress management techniques. Additionally, more research is needed to fully understand the effectiveness, optimal dosages, and long-term safety of these supplements.

# Chapter 4: Optimizing Hormonal Health

Hormonal health plays a vital role in our overall well-being and functioning. Hormones are chemical messengers that regulate various bodily processes, including metabolism, growth and development, reproduction, mood, and energy levels. Optimizing hormonal health involves maintaining a balance of hormones and supporting their proper function. In this chapter, we will explore key strategies for optimizing hormonal health, including lifestyle modifications, dietary considerations, stress management, exercise, and sleep.

## 1. Lifestyle Modifications for Hormonal Health

### ➢ *Stress Management:*

Chronic stress can disrupt hormone balance and lead to hormonal imbalances. Implement stress management techniques such as mindfulness meditation, deep breathing exercises, yoga, or engaging in hobbies and activities that promote relaxation. Finding healthy outlets to manage stress is crucial for maintaining optimal hormonal health.

### ➢ *Adequate Sleep:*

Quality sleep is essential for hormone regulation. Aim for 7-8 hours of uninterrupted sleep each night. Create a sleep-friendly environment, establish a consistent sleep schedule, and practice good sleep hygiene to promote restful sleep and support hormonal balance.

➢ *Regular Exercise:*

Engaging in regular physical activity has numerous benefits for hormonal health. Exercise helps regulate hormone levels, improve insulin sensitivity, promote weight management, and reduce stress. Aim for a combination of cardiovascular exercise, strength training, and flexibility exercises to support overall hormonal balance.

➢ *Weight Management:*

Maintaining a healthy weight is important for hormonal health. Excess body fat, particularly around the abdomen, can lead to hormonal imbalances, such as insulin resistance and increased estrogen levels. Focus on a balanced diet, regular exercise, and portion control to achieve and maintain a healthy weight.

## 2. Dietary Considerations for Hormonal Health

➢ *Balanced Diet:*

Follow a balanced diet that includes a variety of whole foods. Include lean proteins, whole grains, fruits, vegetables, healthy fats, and adequate fiber. A well-rounded diet provides essential nutrients that support hormone production and function.

➢ *Nutrient-Dense Foods:*

Incorporate foods rich in nutrients that support hormonal health. Examples include fatty fish (rich in omega-3 fatty acids), nuts and seeds (rich in healthy fats and minerals), cruciferous vegetables (such as broccoli and cauliflower), berries (rich in antioxidants), and fermented foods (such as yogurt and sauerkraut).

➢ *Healthy Fats:*

Include healthy fats in your diet, such as avocados, olive oil, nuts, and seeds. Healthy fats provide essential fatty acids that support hormone production and absorption. Avoid Tran's fats and limit saturated fats, as they can contribute to inflammation and hormonal imbalances.

➢ *Fiber-Rich Foods:*

Consuming adequate fiber is important for hormonal health. High-fiber foods help regulate blood sugar levels, promote healthy digestion, and support weight management. Include sources of fiber such as whole grains, fruits, vegetables, legumes, and nuts in your diet.

## 3. Hormonal Health and Stress Management

➢ *Stress Reduction Techniques:*

Implement stress management techniques to reduce the impact of chronic stress on hormone balance. Engage in activities that promote relaxation, such as mindfulness meditation, deep breathing exercises, yoga, or spending time in nature. Find healthy outlets to manage stress and prioritize self-care.

➢ *Mind-Body Practices:*

Practices like mindfulness meditation, tai chi, or qigong can promote relaxation and balance the stress response. These practices have been shown to reduce cortisol levels, improve mood, and support overall hormonal health.

➢ *Social Support:*

Maintaining social connections and seeking support from friends, family, or support groups can help reduce stress levels. Sharing feelings and experiences with others can provide emotional support and help manage stress more effectively.

## 4. Exercise and Hormonal Health

Regular Exercise RoutineRegular exercise is beneficial for hormonal health. It helps regulate hormone levels, improve insulin sensitivity, promote weight management, and reduce stress. Aim for a combination of cardiovascular exercise, strength training, and flexibility exercises to support overall hormonal balance.

➤ *Resistance Training:*

Incorporate resistance training into your exercise routine. Resistance exercises, such as weightlifting or bodyweight exercises, promote muscle growth and strength. Increased muscle mass is associated with higher testosterone levels in both men and women.

➤ *High-Intensity Interval Training (HIIT):*

Include HIIT workouts in your exercise regimen. HIIT involves short bursts of intense exercise followed by brief recovery periods. HIIT has been shown to stimulate testosterone production and provide metabolic benefits. It can also help reduce insulin resistance and improve cardiovascular health.

➤ *Endurance Training:*

Engage in moderate-intensity endurance exercises, such as running, cycling, or swimming. Moderate-intensity endurance training has been found to have positive effects on hormonal health, particularly in untrained individuals. However, avoid excessive training loads and allow for adequate rest and recovery.

## 5. Optimizing Sleep for Hormonal Health

➤ *Prioritize Sufficient Sleep Duration:*

Ensure that you are getting enough sleep on a regular basis. Aim for 7-8 hours of uninterrupted sleep each night. Sufficient sleep duration supports hormone regulation, including the production and balance of various hormones.

## ➢ *Establish a Consistent Sleep Schedule:*

Maintain a regular sleep routine by going to bed and waking up at the same time each day, even on weekends. This helps regulate the body's internal clock and promotes better sleep quality.

## ➢ *Create a Sleep-Friendly Environment:*

Ensure that your bedroom is conducive to sleep. Create a cool, dark, and quiet environment that promotes relaxation. Use blackout curtains, earplugs, or white noise machines if necessary. Remove electronic devices that emit blue light, as this can interfere with sleep.

## ➢ *Practice Relaxation Techniques Before Bed:*

Engage in activities that promote relaxation before bedtime. This can include reading a book, taking a warm bath, practicing relaxation exercises, or listening to calming music. Avoid stimulating activities or bright screens close to bedtime.

Optimizing hormonal health is crucial for overall well-being and vitality. Lifestyle modifications, including stress management, regular exercise, healthy eating habits, and sufficient sleep, play significant roles in supporting hormone balance. By implementing these strategies, individuals can promote optimal hormonal health, reduce the risk of hormonal imbalances, and improve their overall quality of life. It is important to prioritize hormonal health as an integral part of a comprehensive approach to wellness.

## 4.1 Understanding the Endocrine System

The endocrine system is a complex network of glands and hormones that work together to regulate various bodily functions. It plays a vital role in maintaining homeostasis, growth, development, reproduction, metabolism, and overall well-being. In this article, we will explore the components of the endocrine system, the major glands and hormones involved, their functions, and the importance of hormonal balance for optimal health.

### 1. Anatomy and Components of the Endocrine System

➢ *Glands:*

The endocrine system consists of several glands located throughout the body. These glands are responsible for producing and secreting hormones into the bloodstream. Major endocrine glands include the pituitary gland, thyroid gland, adrenal glands, pancreas, ovaries (in females), and testes (in males).

➢ *Hormones:*

Hormones are chemical messengers produced by endocrine glands. They travel through the bloodstream and bind to specific receptors in target cells or tissues, initiating various physiological responses. Hormones regulate numerous bodily functions, including growth and development, metabolism, reproduction, and mood.

## 2. Major Glands and Their Hormones

➢ *Pituitary Gland:*

Often referred to as the "master gland," the pituitary gland is located at the base of the brain. It produces and releases several hormones that regulate other endocrine glands, including growth hormone (GH), thyroid-stimulating hormone (TSH), adrenocorticotropic hormone (ACTH), follicle-stimulating hormone (FSH), luteinizing hormone (LH), and prolactin.

➢ *Thyroid Gland:*

The thyroid gland is located in the neck and produces thyroid hormones, primarily thyroxine (T4) and triiodothyronine (T3). These hormones regulate metabolism, growth, and development. The thyroid gland is controlled by the pituitary gland through the release of TSH.

➢ *Adrenal Glands:*

The adrenal glands are situated on top of the kidneys. They produce several hormones, including cortisol, which regulates stress response and metabolism, and aldosterone, which helps regulate blood pressure and electrolyte balance. The adrenal glands also produce adrenaline and noradrenaline, which are involved in the "fight or flight" response.

➢ *Pancreas:*

The pancreas is an organ located behind the stomach. It plays a dual role as an endocrine and exocrine gland. The endocrine part of the pancreas produces hormones such as insulin, which regulates blood sugar levels, and glucagon, which helps increase blood sugar levels. These hormones play a crucial role in glucose metabolism.

➢ *Ovaries and Testes:*

The ovaries, located in the female reproductive system, produce hormones such as estrogen and progesterone, which regulate menstrual cycles and support pregnancy. In males, the testes produce testosterone, the primary male sex hormone responsible for male reproductive development and sexual characteristics.

## 3. Hormonal Regulation and Feedback Mechanisms

➢ *Negative Feedback:*

Hormonal regulation in the endocrine system often operates through negative feedback loops. In a negative feedback loop, the release of a hormone is inhibited or reduced in response to high levels of the hormone. This helps maintain hormonal balance and prevent excessive hormone production.

> ***Hypothalamus-Pituitary Axis:***

The hypothalamus, located in the brain, plays a crucial role in controlling the release of hormones from the pituitary gland. It produces releasing and inhibiting hormones that travel to the pituitary gland and stimulate or suppress the release of specific hormones. This axis is essential for maintaining hormonal balance and coordinating the activities of other endocrine glands.

## 4. Importance of Hormonal Balance

> ***Homeostasis:***

Hormonal balance is crucial for maintaining homeostasis in the body. Hormones work together to regulate various physiological processes and ensure that internal conditions remain stable. Imbalances in hormone levels can lead to disruptions in bodily functions and health issues.

> ***Growth and Development:***

Hormones play a vital role in growth and development, especially during childhood and adolescence. Growth hormones, thyroid hormones, and sex hormones are essential for proper bone growth, muscle development, and sexual maturation.

> ***Metabolism and Energy Regulation:***

Hormones, such as insulin, thyroid hormones, and cortisol, regulate metabolism and energy balance. They influence the breakdown, storage, and utilization of nutrients, including carbohydrates, fats, and proteins. Hormonal imbalances can lead to metabolic disorders, weight gain or loss, and altered energy levels.

> ***Reproduction and Fertility:***

Sex hormones, including estrogen, progesterone, and testosterone, are critical for reproductive health and fertility. They regulate the menstrual cycle, ovulation, sperm production, and the development of secondary sexual characteristics. Hormonal imbalances can disrupt reproductive function and fertility.

> ***Mood and Emotional Well-being:***

Hormones, including serotonin, dopamine, and oxytocin, play a role in regulating mood, emotions, and mental well-being. Imbalances in these hormones can contribute to mood disorders such as depression, anxiety, and mood swings.

*➢ Stress Response:*

Hormones such as cortisol and adrenaline are involved in the body's response to stress. They help mobilize energy, increase heart rate, and prepare the body for action. Chronic stress and dysregulation of stress hormones can have detrimental effects on overall health and well-being.

The endocrine system is a complex network of glands and hormones that regulate various bodily functions. It plays a vital role in maintaining homeostasis, growth, development, reproduction, metabolism, and overall well-being. Understanding the components of the endocrine system, the major glands and hormones involved, and the importance of hormonal balance is crucial for maintaining optimal health. Hormonal imbalances can lead to a wide range of health issues, so it is essential to prioritize hormonal health and seek medical attention if any imbalances or concerns arise.

## 4.2 Balancing Hormones for Optimal Performance

Hormones play a crucial role in regulating various bodily functions, including metabolism, growth, energy levels, mood, and overall performance. Achieving and maintaining hormonal balance is essential for optimal physical and mental performance. In this article, we will explore strategies for balancing hormones to enhance performance, including lifestyle modifications, dietary considerations, stress management, exercise, and adequate rest.

## 1. Lifestyle Modifications for Hormonal Balance

> ➤ *Stress Management:*

Chronic stress can disrupt hormone balance and negatively impact performance. Implement stress management techniques such as mindfulness meditation, deep breathing exercises, yoga, or engaging in activities that promote relaxation. Finding healthy outlets to manage stress is crucial for maintaining optimal hormonal balance.

> ➤ *Adequate Sleep:*

Quality sleep is essential for hormone regulation and performance. Aim for 7-8 hours of uninterrupted sleep each night. Create a sleep-friendly environment, establish a consistent sleep schedule, and practice good sleep hygiene to promote restful sleep and support hormonal balance.

> ➤ *Healthy Weight Management:*

Maintaining a healthy weight is important for hormonal balance and performance. Excess body fat, particularly around the abdomen, can lead to hormonal imbalances and decreased performance. Focus on a balanced diet, regular exercise, and portion control to achieve and maintain a healthy weight.

## 2. Dietary Considerations for Hormonal Balance

➢ *Balanced Diet:*

Follow a balanced diet that includes a variety of whole foods. Include lean proteins, whole grains, fruits, vegetables, healthy fats, and adequate fiber. A well-rounded diet provides essential nutrients that support hormone production and function.

➢ *Healthy Fats:*

Include healthy fats in your diet, such as avocados, olive oil, nuts, and seeds. Healthy fats provide essential fatty acids that support hormone production and absorption. Avoid trans fats and limit saturated fats, as they can contribute to inflammation and hormonal imbalances.

➢ *Protein-Rich Foods:*

Ensure an adequate intake of high-quality proteins, as they are essential for hormone synthesis and repair of tissues. Include sources such as lean meats, fish, poultry, eggs, dairy products, legumes, and plant-based proteins.

➢ *Limit Sugar and Processed Foods:*

Excessive consumption of sugar and processed foods can lead to insulin resistance and hormonal imbalances. Limit your intake of sugary beverages, refined carbohydrates, and processed foods high in unhealthy fats and additives. Instead, focus on whole, unprocessed foods to support hormonal balance.

## 3. Stress Management and Hormonal Balance

➢ *Regular Exercise:*

Engaging in regular physical activity has numerous benefits for hormonal balance. Exercise helps regulate hormone levels, reduce stress, improve mood, and enhance overall performance. Incorporate a combination of cardiovascular exercise, strength training, and flexibility exercises into your routine.

➢ *Mind-Body Practices:*

Practices such as mindfulness meditation, tai chi, or yoga can help reduce stress levels and support hormonal balance. These practices have been shown to reduce cortisol levels, improve mood, and enhance overall well-being.

➢ *Social Support:*

Maintaining social connections and seeking support from friends, family, or support groups can help reduce stress levels. Sharing feelings and experiences with others can provide emotional support and help manage stress more effectively.

## 4. Exercise and Hormonal Balance

➤ *Resistance Training:*

Incorporate resistance training into your exercise routine. Resistance exercises, such as weightlifting or bodyweight exercises, promote muscle growth and strength. Increased muscle mass is associated with higher testosterone levels, which can enhance performance.

➤ *High-Intensity Interval Training (HIIT):*

Include HIIT workouts in your exercise regimen. HIIT involves short bursts of intense exercise followed by brief recovery periods. HIIT has been shown to stimulate hormone production and provide metabolic benefits. It can also help reduce insulin resistance and improve cardiovascular health.

➤ *Endurance Training:*

Engage in moderate-intensity endurance exercises, such as running, cycling, or swimming. Moderate-intensity endurance training has been found to have positive effects on hormonal balance, particularly in untrained individuals. However, avoid excessive training loads and allow for adequate rest and recovery.

Balancing hormones is crucial for optimal performance, both physically and mentally. Lifestyle modifications, including stress management, adequate sleep, and maintaining a healthy weight, play a significant role in achieving hormonal balance. Additionally, dietary considerations, such as consuming a balanced diet rich in healthy fats and proteins while limiting sugar and processed foods, support hormone production and function. Engaging in regular exercise, including resistance training and HIIT, can further optimize hormonal balance and enhance performance. By implementing these strategies, individuals can achieve and maintain optimal hormonal balance, leading to improved overall performance and well-being. It is important to prioritize hormonal health as an integral part of a comprehensive approach to achieving peak performance.

## 4.3 The Impact of Environmental Factors on Hormonal Health

Hormonal health plays a critical role in maintaining overall well-being and proper bodily functions. However, hormonal balance can be influenced by various environmental factors. In this article, we will explore the impact of environmental factors on hormonal health, including exposure to chemicals, pollutants, lifestyle choices, and the importance of creating a hormone-friendly environment.

1.  **Endocrine Disrupting Chemicals (EDCs)**

> *Definition and Sources:*

Endocrine-disrupting chemicals (EDCs) are substances that interfere with the normal functioning of the endocrine system, including hormone production, release, transport, and binding. Common sources of EDCs include pesticides, industrial chemicals, plasticizers, and personal care products.

> ***Examples of EDCs:***

- Bisphenol A (BPA): Found in plastic containers, food can linings, and thermal paper receipts. It has been linked to hormonal imbalances and reproductive health issues.
- Phthalates: Used in plastics, cosmetics, and fragrances. Phthalates have been associated with adverse effects on reproductive health and hormone disruption.
- Organochlorine pesticides: Chemicals such as DDT and dioxins have been linked to hormone-related disorders and reproductive problems.

> ***Health Effects of EDCs:***

EDCs can disrupt hormonal balance and contribute to various health issues, including infertility, reproductive disorders, developmental abnormalities, thyroid dysfunction, and increased risk of certain cancers. The effects can be particularly significant during prenatal and early childhood development.

## 2. Air and Water Pollution

> ***Air Pollution:***

Exposure to air pollutants, such as particulate matter, volatile organic compounds (VOCs), and nitrogen dioxide, has been associated with hormonal disruptions. Air pollution has been linked to increased risks of respiratory diseases, cardiovascular issues, and hormonal imbalances.

➢ *Water Pollution:*

Contamination of water sources with EDCs, pharmaceuticals, and industrial chemicals can pose a risk to hormonal health. Chemicals like perchlorates and pharmaceutical residues in water supplies have been shown to interfere with thyroid hormone function.

## 3. Lifestyle Choices and Hormonal Health

➢ *Diet and Nutrition:*

Unhealthy dietary choices, such as a diet high in processed foods, unhealthy fats, and added sugars, can contribute to hormonal imbalances. Nutrient deficiencies, particularly in vitamins and minerals essential for hormone production and function, can also impact hormonal health.

➢ *Physical Activity:*

A sedentary lifestyle and lack of regular exercise can affect hormonal balance. Regular physical activity has been associated with improved

insulin sensitivity, reduced cortisol levels, and better hormonal
regulation.

> ***Stress and Emotional Well-being:***

Chronic stress can disrupt hormonal balance and contribute to a range of
health issues. Elevated cortisol levels, resulting from prolonged stress,
can impact other hormone levels and lead to adrenal fatigue or
dysregulation.

## 4. Creating a Hormone-Friendly Environment

> ***Reduce Exposure to EDCs:***

Minimize exposure to EDCs by choosing products labeled as BPA-free,
using natural and organic personal care products, and opting for organic
foods. Be cautious of food and drink containers made from plastics or
cans with potential BPA linings.

> ***Indoor Air Quality:***

Improve indoor air quality by reducing exposure to indoor pollutants.
Use air purifiers, ensure proper ventilation, and avoid smoking or
exposure to secondhand smoke.

➢ *Water Filtration:*

Invest in a high-quality water filtration system to remove contaminants from tap water, including EDCs and other chemicals that can disrupt hormonal balance.

➢ *Healthy Lifestyle Choices:*

Adopt a healthy lifestyle that includes a balanced diet, regular exercise, stress management techniques, and adequate sleep. These practices support hormonal health and overall well-being.

Environmental factors have a significant impact on hormonal health. Exposure to endocrine-disrupting chemicals, air and water pollution, and lifestyle choices can disrupt hormonal balance and contribute to various health issues. It is crucial to be aware of potential sources of exposure, make informed choices regarding products and lifestyle habits, and create a hormone-friendly environment. By minimizing exposure to EDCs, reducing air and water pollution, and adopting healthy lifestyle choices, individuals can support optimal hormonal health and improve their overall well-being.

# Chapter 5: Lifestyle Strategies for Peak Performance

Peak performance refers to achieving and maintaining optimal physical and mental abilities to excel in various areas of life. Lifestyle plays a crucial role in supporting peak performance. In this chapter, we will explore key lifestyle strategies that can enhance performance, including nutrition, hydration, sleep, stress management, and goal setting.

## 1. Nutrition for Peak Performance

➤ *Balanced Diet:*

A balanced diet is essential for providing the necessary nutrients to support optimal performance. Include a variety of fruits, vegetables, whole grains, lean proteins, and healthy fats. Prioritize nutrient-dense foods that provide sustained energy and promote overall health.

➤ *Macronutrient Distribution:*

Ensure appropriate distribution of macronutrients for energy and muscle recovery. Consume adequate carbohydrates for fuel, sufficient protein for muscle repair and growth, and healthy fats for energy and hormonal balance.

➤ *Meal Timing:*

Consider the timing of meals to support performance. Fuel your body with a balanced meal or snack before workouts or competitions. Additionally, post-workout nutrition is crucial for replenishing glycogen stores and aiding in muscle recovery.

➢ *Hydration:*

Proper hydration is vital for optimal performance. Drink water regularly throughout the day, and increase fluid intake during physical activity. Pay attention to signs of dehydration and adjust fluid intake accordingly.

## 2. Sleep for Peak Performance

➢ *Sleep Duration:*

Prioritize sufficient sleep for optimal performance. Aim for 7-9 hours of quality sleep each night. Individual sleep needs may vary, so listen to your body and adjust sleep duration accordingly.

➢ *Sleep Environment:*

Create a sleep-friendly environment to promote restful sleep. Keep your bedroom cool, dark, and quiet. Remove electronic devices and establish a relaxing pre-sleep routine to signal to your body that it's time to rest.

➢ *Consistent Sleep Schedule:*

Maintain a regular sleep schedule by going to bed and waking up at the same time each day, even on weekends. Consistency helps regulate the body's internal clock and promotes better sleep quality.

## 3. Stress Management for Peak Performance

➢ *Stress Awareness:*

Recognize and manage stress to optimize performance. Identify stressors and develop strategies to cope with them effectively. Practice mindfulness, deep breathing exercises, or engage in activities that promote relaxation and stress reduction.

➢ *Time Management:*

Effectively manage time to minimize stress and maximize productivity. Prioritize tasks, set realistic goals, and allocate time for rest and relaxation. Break down larger tasks into smaller, manageable steps to reduce stress and increase focus.

➢ *Self-Care:*

Make self-care a priority to support peak performance. Engage in activities that promote mental and emotional well-being, such as hobbies, exercise, socializing, or spending time in nature. Take breaks when needed and practice self-compassion.

## 4. Goal Setting for Peak Performance

> ### *SMART Goals:*

Set specific, measurable, achievable, relevant, and time-bound (SMART) goals. Clearly define what you want to achieve and establish a plan of action to reach your goals. Break larger goals into smaller milestones for a sense of progress and motivation.

> ### *Visualization and Positive Thinking:*

Use visualization techniques to imagine yourself successfully achieving your goals. Positive thinking and self-belief can enhance motivation and performance. Cultivate a growth mindset and focus on the process of improvement.

> ### *Accountability and Support:*

Seek accountability and support from others to stay motivated and on track. Share your goals with a trusted friend, coach, or mentor who can provide guidance, encouragement, and feedback.

Lifestyle strategies play a vital role in supporting peak performance. Nutrition, hydration, sleep, stress management, and goal setting are key components of an effective lifestyle approach. By adopting these strategies, individuals can optimize their physical and mental abilities, enhance performance, and achieve their goals. Remember that everyone is unique, so it's important to personalize these strategies to suit your individual needs and preferences. Prioritize your well-being, make intentional choices, and strive for a balanced and healthy lifestyle to reach your peak performance potential.

## 5.1 Strategies for Maintaining a Healthy Weight

Maintaining a healthy weight is essential for overall health and well-being. It helps reduce the risk of chronic diseases, enhances energy levels, and improves quality of life. In this chapter, we will explore strategies for maintaining a healthy weight, including adopting a balanced diet, engaging in regular physical activity, managing portion sizes, practicing mindful eating, and building a supportive environment.

### 1. Balanced Diet for Weight Maintenance

➢ *Caloric Balance:*

Achieve a balance between calorie intake and expenditure. Monitor your calorie intake by being aware of portion sizes and choosing nutrient-dense foods. Avoid excessive calorie consumption, as it can lead to weight gain.

➢ *Nutrient-Rich Foods:*

Emphasize nutrient-rich foods in your diet, including fruits, vegetables, whole grains, lean proteins, and healthy fats. These foods provide essential nutrients while keeping you satisfied and supporting overall health.

➢ *Portion Control:*

Be mindful of portion sizes to avoid overeating. Use smaller plates, bowls, and utensils to create the perception of a fuller plate. Pay attention to hunger and fullness cues, and avoid eating until you feel uncomfortably full.

➢ *Regular Meals and Snacks:*

Establish regular meal and snack times to maintain stable blood sugar levels and prevent excessive hunger. Avoid skipping meals, as it can lead to overeating later in the day. Include a balance of macronutrients (carbohydrates, proteins, and fats) in each meal to promote satiety.

## 2. Regular Physical Activity for Weight Maintenance

➢ *Aerobic Exercise:*

Engage in regular aerobic activities such as walking, jogging, swimming, or cycling. Aim for at least 150 minutes of moderate-intensity aerobic exercise or 75 minutes of vigorous-intensity exercise per week. This helps burn calories, maintain muscle mass, and support weight management.

> ➤ *Strength Training:*

Incorporate strength training exercises into your routine to build and maintain muscle mass. Muscles burn more calories than fat, even at rest, so increasing muscle mass can support weight management. Include exercises that target all major muscle groups at least twice a week.

> ➤ *Active Lifestyle:*

Adopt an active lifestyle by incorporating physical activity into your daily routine. Take the stairs instead of the elevator, walk or bike instead of driving short distances, and find activities you enjoy that keep you moving throughout the day.

### 3. Mindful Eating and Behavior Modification

> ➤ *Mindful Eating:*

Practice mindful eating by paying attention to your food choices, eating slowly, and savoring each bite. Be aware of hunger and fullness cues, and eat until you are comfortably satisfied, not overly full. Minimize distractions while eating, such as television or electronic devices.

> ### *Emotional Eating:*

Recognize and address emotional eating triggers. Develop alternative coping mechanisms for dealing with emotions, such as engaging in hobbies, practicing relaxation techniques, or seeking support from friends and family.

> ### *Self-Monitoring:*

Keep a food diary or use a mobile app to track your food intake. This helps create awareness of your eating patterns and provides insight into your calorie consumption. It can also help identify areas for improvement and promote accountability.

> ### *Behavior Modification Techniques:*

Implement behavior modification techniques to support healthy eating habits. Set realistic goals, reward yourself for achievements, and create a supportive environment by removing tempting foods and surrounding yourself with positive influences.

## 4. Building a Supportive Environment

➢ *Social Support:*

Surround yourself with a supportive network of friends, family, or a weight management group. Engaging in activities together, sharing experiences, and providing encouragement can help you stay motivated and accountable.

➢ *Healthy Food Environment:*

Create a healthy food environment at home by stocking your pantry and refrigerator with nutritious foods. Limit the presence of unhealthy snacks and sugary beverages, making healthier choices more accessible.

➢ *Meal Preparation:*

Plan and prepare meals in advance to avoid relying on convenience foods or ordering takeout. Meal prepping allows you to control portion sizes, make healthier choices, and save time and money.

➢ *Sleep and Stress Management:*

Prioritize sufficient sleep and practice stress management techniques. Inadequate sleep and chronic stress can disrupt appetite-regulating hormones and contribute to weight gain. Aim for 7-9 hours of quality sleep and engage in stress-reducing activities such as meditation, yoga, or deep breathing exercises.

Maintaining a healthy weight requires a combination of healthy eating habits, regular physical activity, mindful eating, behavior modification, and a supportive environment. By adopting these strategies, individuals can achieve and sustain a healthy weight, improve overall health, and enhance their quality of life. Remember that weight management is a journey, and small, sustainable changes are key to long-term success.

## 5.2 Building Lean Muscle Mass and Strength Training

Building lean muscle mass and increasing strength is not only important for athletes and bodybuilders but also for individuals looking to improve their overall health and physique. In this chapter, we will explore the principles and strategies behind building lean muscle mass through strength training. We will cover topics such as the benefits of strength training, the principles of muscle hypertrophy, designing an effective strength training program, nutrition for muscle growth, and recovery strategies.

### 1. Benefits of Strength Training

➢ *Increased Muscle Mass:*

Strength training stimulates muscle hypertrophy, leading to an increase in lean muscle mass. More muscle mass not only improves strength and athletic performance but also boosts metabolism, aiding in weight management.

➢ *Improved Strength and Power:*

Strength training enhances muscular strength and power, allowing individuals to perform daily tasks with ease and excel in athletic pursuits.

➢ *Enhanced Bone Health:*

Resistance training contributes to improved bone mineral density, reducing the risk of osteoporosis and fractures.

➢ *Metabolic Health:*

Strength training improves insulin sensitivity and glucose metabolism, contributing to better blood sugar control and reducing the risk of type 2 diabetes.

## 2. Principles of Muscle Hypertrophy

➢ *Progressive Overload:*

To stimulate muscle growth, progressively increase the demands placed on the muscles over time. This can be achieved by increasing resistance (weight), repetitions, or training volume.

### ➤ *Specificity:*

Adapt your training program to target the specific muscles or muscle groups you want to develop. Choose exercises that target those muscles and perform them with proper form and technique.

### ➤ *Volume and Frequency:*

Aim for an optimal balance of training volume (total sets, reps, and resistance) and training frequency (how often you train a muscle group). Gradually increase both volume and frequency as your body adapts to the training stimulus.

### ➤ *Variation:*

Incorporate variety into your training program to prevent plateaus and keep the muscles challenged. This can include changing exercises, manipulating rep ranges, or using different training techniques.

## 3. Designing an Effective Strength Training Program

### ➤ *Exercise Selection:*

Choose compound exercises that engage multiple muscle groups, such as squats, deadlifts, bench presses, and overhead presses. These exercises provide a strong foundation for overall muscle development.

➤ *Repetition Range:*

To promote muscle hypertrophy, perform exercises in a moderate to high repetition range (around 8-12 reps per set). This range optimizes both muscle fiber recruitment and metabolic stress.

➤ *Sets and Rest Periods:*

Perform 3-5 sets per exercise, allowing for adequate rest between sets (typically 1-3 minutes) to maximize recovery and maintain intensity.

➤ *Training Frequency:*

Train each muscle group 2-3 times per week, allowing for adequate recovery between sessions. Splitting your workouts into different muscle groups on different days can help distribute the workload and prevent overtraining.

## 4. Nutrition for Muscle Growth

➤ *Caloric Surplus:*

To support muscle growth, consume a slight caloric surplus by eating more calories than your body requires for maintenance. This provides the energy and nutrients needed for muscle repair and growth.

➢ *Protein Intake:*

Ensure an adequate protein intake to support muscle synthesis. Aim for 1.6-2.2 grams of protein per kilogram of body weight per day, distributing it evenly throughout your meals.

➢ *Carbohydrates and Fats:*

Include carbohydrates for energy and replenishing glycogen stores, and healthy fats for hormone production and overall health. Choose complex carbohydrates and prioritize sources of unsaturated fats.

➢ *Meal Timing:*

Distribute your protein and calorie intake evenly throughout the day to support muscle protein synthesis. Aim for a combination of protein, carbohydrates, and fats in each meal and snack.

## 5. Recovery Strategies

➢ *Rest and Sleep:*

Allow sufficient time for rest and recovery between workouts. Aim for 48-72 hours of rest for each muscle group. Prioritize quality sleep to support muscle repair and growth.

➢ *Active Recovery:*

Engage in light physical activity or low-intensity exercises on rest days to promote blood flow, reduce muscle soreness, and aid in recovery.

➢ *Stretching and Mobility:*

Incorporate stretching and mobility exercises into your routine to maintain flexibility, prevent injuries, and improve muscle function.

➢ *Hydration and Nutrition:*

Stay hydrated throughout the day to support optimal muscle function and recovery. Consume a balanced diet with adequate protein, carbohydrates, and fats to provide the necessary nutrients for recovery.

Building lean muscle mass and increasing strength requires a combination of progressive overload, proper nutrition, and adequate recovery. By following the principles of muscle hypertrophy, designing an effective strength training program, fueling your body with the right nutrients, and prioritizing recovery, you can achieve your muscle-building goals and improve your overall physical performance. Remember to listen to your body, adjust your program as needed, and seek guidance from a qualified fitness professional if necessary.

## 5.3 Mental and Emotional Well-being for Optimal Hormonal Balance

Optimal hormonal balance is crucial for overall health and well-being. While physical factors play a significant role, mental and emotional well-being also greatly impact hormonal balance. In this chapter, we will explore the connection between mental and emotional health and hormonal balance, and discuss strategies for cultivating a positive mindset, managing stress, promoting emotional well-being, and fostering a healthy hormonal environment.

### 1. The Mind-Body Connection

➤ *Understanding Hormonal Balance:*

Hormones play a vital role in regulating various bodily functions, including metabolism, mood, sleep, and reproductive health. Imbalances in hormone levels can lead to a range of physical and emotional symptoms.

➤ *Stress and Hormonal Imbalance:*

Chronic stress can disrupt the delicate balance of hormones in the body. Stress hormones, such as cortisol, can interfere with the production and regulation of other hormones, leading to imbalances.

## 2. Cultivating a Positive Mindset

### ➢ *Positive Thinking and Self-Talk:*

Practice positive thinking and self-talk to cultivate a positive mindset. Challenge negative thoughts and replace them with positive and empowering affirmations.

### ➢ *Gratitude Practice:*

Engage in a gratitude practice by expressing gratitude for the things you appreciate in your life. This practice can help shift your focus to the positive aspects and increase overall well-being.

### ➢ *Mindfulness and Meditation:*

Incorporate mindfulness and meditation into your daily routine. These practices can help reduce stress, improve focus, and promote a sense of calm and balance.

## 3. Managing Stress for Hormonal Balance

### ➢ *Stress Reduction Techniques:*

Explore various stress reduction techniques such as deep breathing exercises, yoga, tai chi, or engaging in hobbies and activities that bring you joy. Find what works best for you and make it a regular part of your routine.

> ***Time Management and Prioritization:***

Manage your time effectively and prioritize tasks to reduce feelings of overwhelm and stress. Break down tasks into smaller, manageable steps, and delegate or seek support when needed.

> ***Setting Boundaries:***

Establish healthy boundaries in your personal and professional life. Learn to say no when necessary, and prioritize self-care and activities that promote relaxation and stress relief.

## 4. Emotional Well-being and Hormonal Balance

> ***Social Support:***

Cultivate strong social connections and seek support from friends, family, or support groups. Having a supportive network can help reduce stress, improve mood, and promote emotional well-being.

> *Healthy Relationships:*

Foster healthy and positive relationships in your life. Surround yourself with people who uplift and support you, and engage in open and honest communication to maintain healthy connections.

> *Emotional Expression and Processing:*

Find healthy outlets for expressing and processing emotions, such as journaling, art, or talking to a trusted friend or therapist. Acknowledge and validate your emotions, and practice self-compassion.

## 5. Lifestyle Habits for Hormonal Balance

> *Regular Physical Activity:*

Engage in regular exercise to boost mood, reduce stress, and support hormonal balance. Find activities that you enjoy and make them a part of your routine.

> *Healthy Sleep Habits:*

Prioritize quality sleep to support hormonal balance. Establish a consistent sleep schedule, create a relaxing bedtime routine, and create a sleep-friendly environment.

> *Balanced Nutrition:*

Maintain a balanced diet rich in nutrient-dense foods to support overall health and hormonal balance. Include foods that support hormone production, such as omega-3 fatty acids, antioxidants, and fiber.

Mental and emotional well-being is essential for maintaining optimal hormonal balance. By cultivating a positive mindset, managing stress effectively, promoting emotional well-being, and adopting healthy lifestyle habits, individuals can create a harmonious environment for their hormones to thrive. Remember that everyone's journey is unique, and it's important to seek support from healthcare professionals or therapists if needed. Prioritize self-care, embrace positive habits, and nurture your mental and emotional well-being for a healthier hormonal balance.

# Chapter 6: Long-Term Hormonal Health and Vitality

Maintaining long-term hormonal health and vitality is crucial for overall well-being and quality of life. Hormones play a significant role in regulating various bodily functions, including metabolism, reproduction, mood, and energy levels. In this chapter, we will explore the key factors and strategies for promoting long-term hormonal health and vitality. We will discuss the importance of regular check-ups, the impact of lifestyle choices, the role of hormone replacement therapy, and the significance of mental and emotional well-being.

## 1. Regular Hormonal Check-ups

### ➢ *Understanding Hormonal Changes:*

Regular hormonal check-ups help monitor hormone levels and detect any imbalances or abnormalities. Understanding the natural hormonal changes that occur with age and other factors can guide the monitoring process.

### ➢ *Hormone Testing:*

Regular hormone testing, including blood tests and other diagnostic methods, allows healthcare professionals to assess hormone levels and identify any deficiencies or excesses.

➢ *Consultation with Healthcare Professionals:*

Schedule regular consultations with healthcare professionals, such as endocrinologists or hormone specialists, to discuss any concerns, review test results, and develop an individualized plan for long-term hormonal health.

## 2. Lifestyle Choices and Hormonal Health

➢ *Balanced Diet:*

Adopting a balanced diet rich in nutrients, including fruits, vegetables, whole grains, lean proteins, and healthy fats, supports optimal hormonal health. Avoiding excessive sugar, processed foods, and unhealthy fats is essential.

➢ *Regular Exercise:*

Engaging in regular physical activity, including aerobic exercises, strength training, and flexibility exercises, promotes hormonal balance and overall well-being. Aim for a combination of cardiovascular exercises and strength training to support muscle mass and metabolism.

➢ *Stress Management:*

Chronic stress can negatively impact hormone levels. Implement stress management techniques, such as meditation, deep breathing exercises, yoga, or engaging in hobbies, to reduce stress and promote hormonal balance.

> *Adequate Sleep:*

Prioritize sufficient sleep to allow the body to rest and restore hormone levels. Aim for 7-9 hours of quality sleep each night and establish a consistent sleep routine.

> *Avoidance of Harmful Substances:*

Limit or avoid the consumption of harmful substances such as tobacco, excessive alcohol, and recreational drugs. These substances can disrupt hormonal balance and overall health.

## 3. Hormone Replacement Therapy

> *Understanding Hormone Replacement Therapy (HRT):*

HRT is a medical treatment option that involves replacing hormones, such as estrogen, progesterone, or testosterone, to restore hormonal balance. It is commonly used for individuals experiencing hormone deficiencies or imbalances.

 *Consultation with Healthcare Professionals:*

If considering HRT, consult with healthcare professionals specialized in hormone therapy to discuss the potential benefits, risks, and appropriate treatment options tailored to individual needs.

➤ *Monitoring and Adjustments:*

Regular monitoring and evaluation of hormone levels are essential when undergoing HRT. Adjustments to hormone dosage or treatment methods may be necessary to achieve and maintain optimal hormonal balance.

## 4. Mental and Emotional Well-being

➤ *Stress Reduction:*

Manage stress levels through techniques such as mindfulness, meditation, therapy, or engaging in activities that promote relaxation and emotional well-being. Chronic stress can disrupt hormonal balance, so stress reduction is crucial for long-term hormonal health.

➤ *Emotional Support:*

Maintain strong social connections and seek emotional support from friends, family, or support groups. Engaging in open and honest communication can provide emotional stability and contribute to hormonal well-being.

> ➢ *Mental Health Care:*

Prioritize mental health care by seeking therapy or counseling if needed. Addressing and managing underlying mental health conditions, such as anxiety or depression, can positively impact hormonal health.

## 5. Long-Term Lifestyle Habits

> ➢ *Regular Health Screenings:*

Besides hormonal check-ups, schedule regular health screenings, including blood pressure, cholesterol, and diabetes screenings, to monitor the overall health and address any potential concerns.

> ➢ *Preventive Measures:*

Adopt preventive measures such as vaccination, regular dental check-ups, and cancer screenings to maintain overall health and reduce the risk of chronic diseases that can affect hormonal balance.

> ➢ *Healthy Aging:*

Embrace healthy aging practices, including maintaining a positive outlook, engaging in intellectual stimulation, and pursuing hobbies and activities that bring joy and fulfillment.

Promoting long-term hormonal health and vitality requires a holistic approach that encompasses regular check-ups, healthy lifestyle choices, stress management, hormone replacement therapy when necessary, and prioritizing mental and emotional well-being. By taking proactive steps to maintain hormonal balance, individuals can enhance their overall well-being, vitality, and quality of life as they age. Remember to consult with healthcare professionals, make informed choices, and embrace a balanced and healthy lifestyle to support long-term hormonal health and vitality.

## 6.1 Age-Defying Strategies for Sustaining Testosterone Levels

As men age, testosterone levels naturally decline. However, there are strategies that can help sustain testosterone levels and mitigate the effects of age-related decline. In this chapter, we will explore age-defying strategies that focus on lifestyle choices, nutrition, exercise, and overall well-being to support healthy testosterone levels as men grow older.

### 1. Understanding Age-Related Testosterone Decline

➢ *Age-Related Testosterone Changes:*

Explain the natural decline in testosterone levels that occurs with age and how it can impact various aspects of men's health, including energy levels, muscle mass, sexual function, and mood.

> ## *Symptoms of Low Testosterone:*

Discuss the common symptoms of low testosterone, such as fatigue, reduced libido, loss of muscle mass, and mood changes, which can indicate an age-related decline.

## 2. Lifestyle Choices for Sustaining Testosterone Levels

> ## *Regular Physical Activity:*

Highlight the importance of regular exercise, including both cardiovascular exercises and strength training, to stimulate testosterone production and maintain muscle mass.

> ## *Weight Management:*

Explain how maintaining a healthy weight through a balanced diet and regular exercise can help sustain testosterone levels. Discuss the negative impact of obesity on testosterone production.

➢ *Stress Reduction:*

Emphasize the importance of stress management techniques, such as meditation, deep breathing exercises, and engaging in hobbies, to reduce chronic stress and support healthy testosterone levels.

## 3. Nutrition for Testosterone Support

➢ *Balanced Diet:*

Discuss the significance of a balanced diet that includes lean proteins, healthy fats, fruits, vegetables, and whole grains in supporting testosterone production. Highlight specific foods rich in nutrients that support testosterone levels.

➢ *Micronutrients and Supplements:*

Explain the role of specific micronutrients, such as zinc, vitamin D, and magnesium, in testosterone production. Discuss the potential benefits of supplementation in individuals with deficiencies or limited dietary intake.

➢ *Avoidance of Harmful Substances:*

Address the negative impact of excessive alcohol consumption, tobacco use, and certain medications on testosterone levels. Encourage moderation or avoidance of these substances for hormonal health.

### 4. Hormone Optimization Strategies

➢ *Hormone Replacement Therapy (HRT):*

Discuss the option of HRT for individuals with clinically diagnosed low testosterone levels. Explain the benefits, risks, and considerations associated with HRT and the importance of consulting with healthcare professionals.

➢ *Sleep Quality and Duration:*

Highlight the role of quality sleep in supporting testosterone production. Provide tips for improving sleep hygiene and creating a conducive sleep environment.

### 5. Emotional Well-being and Mental Health

➢ *Stress Management:*

Discuss the impact of chronic stress on testosterone levels and highlight stress reduction techniques such as mindfulness, relaxation exercises, and seeking emotional support.

Address the importance of addressing and managing mental health conditions, such as anxiety or depression, which can impact hormonal balance. Encourage seeking professional help when needed.

Maintaining healthy testosterone levels as men age requires a multifaceted approach that includes lifestyle choices, nutrition, exercise, and emotional well-being. By adopting age-defying strategies and making conscious efforts to support testosterone production, men can sustain their vitality, energy levels, muscle mass, and overall well-being. It is essential to consult healthcare professionals, make informed choices, and prioritize self-care to age gracefully and maintain healthy testosterone levels throughout life. Remember that individual responses may vary, and regular monitoring and adjustments may be necessary.

## 6.2 Maintaining Optimal Hormonal Health Beyond 40

As individuals reach the age of 40 and beyond, hormonal changes become more pronounced. Both men and women experience shifts in hormone levels that can affect various aspects of health and well-being. In this chapter, we will explore strategies to maintain optimal hormonal health beyond the age of 40. We will discuss the importance of regular check-ups, lifestyle choices, nutrition, exercise, stress management, and hormone optimization techniques.

### 1. Understanding Hormonal Changes

➢ **Age-Related Hormonal Changes:**

Explain the hormonal changes that occur as individuals age, including menopause in women and andropause in men. Discuss the impact of these changes on hormone levels and overall health.

> ***Common Hormonal Imbalances:***

Highlight common hormonal imbalances that may occur beyond the age of 40, such as estrogen dominance, low testosterone, and thyroid imbalances. Discuss the symptoms and potential consequences of these imbalances.

## 2. Regular Hormonal Check-ups

> ***Importance of Hormonal Testing:***

Emphasize the importance of regular hormonal testing to monitor hormone levels and identify any imbalances or deficiencies. Discuss the different types of tests and the role of healthcare professionals in interpreting the results.

> ***Consultation with Healthcare Professionals:***

Encourage individuals to consult with healthcare professionals, such as endocrinologists or hormone specialists, for guidance on hormonal health beyond 40. Discuss the benefits of personalized treatment plans and ongoing monitoring.

## 3. Lifestyle Choices for Hormonal Health

### ➢ *Balanced Diet:*

Promote the consumption of a balanced diet that includes a variety of nutrient-dense foods. Discuss the importance of macronutrients, such as proteins, healthy fats, and carbohydrates, as well as micronutrients like vitamins and minerals.

### ➢ *Phytoestrogens and Hormonal Balance:*

Explain the role of phytoestrogens, found in foods like soy, flaxseeds, and legumes, in supporting hormonal balance. Discuss the potential benefits of incorporating these foods into the diet.

### ➢ *Alcohol and Caffeine Moderation:*

Highlight the importance of moderating alcohol and caffeine consumption, as excessive intake can disrupt hormonal balance and overall health.

## 4. Exercise and Hormonal Health

### ➢ *Regular Physical Activity:*

Emphasize the benefits of regular exercise for hormonal health, including increased metabolism, improved insulin sensitivity, and enhanced mood. Discuss the importance of a combination of cardiovascular exercises and strength training.

> ***High-Intensity Interval Training (HIIT):***

Introduce the concept of HIIT and its potential benefits for hormonal health, including improved cardiovascular fitness, increased growth hormone production, and enhanced fat metabolism.

## 5. Stress Management for Hormonal Balance

> ***Stress and Hormonal Imbalance:***

Explain the link between chronic stress and hormonal imbalance. Discuss the impact of stress on cortisol levels and its potential consequences for other hormones.

> ***Stress Reduction Techniques:***

Provide various stress reduction techniques, such as mindfulness, meditation, deep breathing exercises, and engaging in hobbies or activities that promote relaxation. Encourage individuals to find what works best for them.

➢ *Work-Life Balance:*

Discuss the importance of establishing a healthy work-life balance to reduce stress levels and support overall hormonal health. Encourage individuals to set boundaries, prioritize self-care, and seek support when needed.

## 6. Hormone Optimization Techniques

➢ *Bioidentical Hormone Replacement Therapy (BHRT):*

Discuss the concept of BHRT, which involves using hormones that are structurally identical to those naturally produced by the body. Explain its potential benefits, risks, and considerations. Highlight the importance of consulting with healthcare professionals.

➢ *Natural Hormone Support:*

Introduce natural approaches to hormone support, such as herbal supplements, adaptogens, and lifestyle modifications. Discuss their potential role in promoting hormonal balance beyond 40.

Maintaining optimal hormonal health beyond the age of 40 requires a multifaceted approach that encompasses regular check-ups, lifestyle choices, nutrition, exercise, stress management, and potentially hormone optimization techniques. By adopting these strategies, individuals can support their hormonal balance, overall well-being, and quality of life as they age. It is crucial to seek guidance from healthcare professionals, make informed choices, and prioritize self-care to achieve and maintain optimal hormonal health beyond 40. Remember that individual needs and responses may vary, so regular monitoring and adjustments may be necessary.


**6.3 Integrating Testosterone Boosting Habits into Daily Life**

Boosting testosterone levels is a goal for many individuals seeking to optimize their health, vitality, and well-being. While there are various approaches to boosting testosterone, integrating specific habits into daily life can provide a sustainable and holistic approach. In this chapter, we will explore practical and actionable habits that can help naturally increase testosterone levels and support overall hormonal health.


## 1. Understanding Testosterone and Its Benefits

> *Importance of Testosterone:*

Explain the role of testosterone in the body, including its impact on muscle mass, bone density, libido, mood, and cognitive function. Discuss the benefits of maintaining optimal testosterone levels.


> *Factors Affecting Testosterone Levels:*

Highlight the various factors, such as age, lifestyle choices, nutrition, exercise, and stress levels, that can influence testosterone production.

Emphasize the importance of addressing these factors for hormonal health.


## 2. Nutrition for Testosterone Support


> ➢ *Balanced Diet:*


Promote the consumption of a balanced diet that includes macronutrients (proteins, healthy fats, and carbohydrates) and micronutrients (vitamins and minerals) necessary for testosterone production. Highlight specific foods that are known to support testosterone levels.


> ➢ *Essential Nutrients for Testosterone:*


Discuss the importance of specific nutrients, such as zinc, vitamin D, magnesium, and omega-3 fatty acids, in supporting testosterone production. Provide practical tips on incorporating these nutrients into daily meals.


> ➢ *Meal Timing and Frequency:*


Explain the potential benefits of meal timing and frequency on testosterone levels. Discuss strategies such as intermittent fasting and regular meals spaced throughout the day.

## 3. Exercise and Testosterone Production

> ### *Resistance Training:*

Highlight the role of resistance training, such as weightlifting and bodyweight exercises, in boosting testosterone levels. Explain the importance of incorporating both compound and isolation exercises into a well-rounded workout routine.

> ### *High-Intensity Interval Training (HIIT):*

Discuss the potential benefits of HIIT workouts in stimulating testosterone production. Explain how short bursts of intense exercise followed by brief recovery periods can be incorporated into daily routines.

> ### *Regular Physical Activity:*

Emphasize the importance of overall physical activity and an active lifestyle in maintaining optimal testosterone levels. Encourage individuals to find activities they enjoy and can sustain long-term.

## 4. Sleep and Stress Management for Hormonal Health

> ### *Quality Sleep:*

Highlight the crucial role of quality sleep in testosterone production and overall hormonal health. Provide tips for improving sleep hygiene and establishing a consistent sleep schedule.

> ➤ *Stress Reduction Techniques:*

Discuss various stress reduction techniques, such as meditation, deep breathing exercises, yoga, and engaging in hobbies, to lower stress levels and support testosterone production.

> ➤ *Prioritizing Relaxation and Self-Care:*

Encourage individuals to prioritize relaxation and self-care activities in their daily routines. This can include activities like taking breaks, practicing mindfulness, and engaging in hobbies or activities that promote relaxation.

## 5. Lifestyle Habits for Testosterone Optimization

> ➤ *Maintaining a Healthy Weight:*

Discuss the impact of excess body fat on testosterone levels and the importance of maintaining a healthy weight through proper nutrition and regular exercise.

➢ *Avoidance of Harmful Substances:*

Highlight the negative effects of excessive alcohol consumption, tobacco use, and drug abuse on testosterone production. Encourage moderation or avoidance of these substances for hormonal health.

➢ *Optimizing Vitamin D Levels:*

Discuss the role of vitamin D in testosterone production and the importance of regular sun exposure or supplementation to maintain optimal vitamin D levels.

Integrating testosterone-boosting habits into daily life is a proactive approach to supporting optimal hormonal health and overall well-being. By focusing on nutrition, exercise, sleep, stress management, and lifestyle choices, individuals can naturally increase testosterone levels and reap the benefits of enhanced vitality, strength, and mental clarity. It is essential to make these habits a consistent part of daily life, seek guidance from healthcare professionals when needed, and listen to the body's signals to ensure long-term success in maintaining healthy testosterone levels. Remember that individual responses may vary, and patience and consistency are key to achieving sustainable results.

# Conclusion

In "The Alpha Formula: The Ultimate Guide to Natural Testosterone Boosting for Men Over 40 at Peak Performance and Elevate Your Hormonal Health and Vitality," we have explored a comprehensive approach to optimizing testosterone levels and achieving peak performance and vitality as men age. Throughout this book, we have delved into the intricacies of testosterone, its importance, and the factors that can affect its levels.

By understanding the changes that occur with age and the impact of lifestyle choices, nutrition, exercise, sleep, stress management, and other factors on testosterone production, readers have gained valuable insights into how to take control of their hormonal health.

We have discussed practical strategies and habits that can be integrated into daily life to naturally boost testosterone levels. From adopting a balanced diet rich in nutrients that support testosterone production to engaging in regular exercise routines that promote muscle strength and overall well-being, readers have learned how to optimize their lifestyles for hormonal health.

Furthermore, we have emphasized the importance of quality sleep, stress management techniques, and relaxation practices to balance hormones and enhance vitality. By addressing these aspects, individuals can cultivate a state of well-being that positively impacts testosterone levels and overall health.

"The Alpha Formula" has also explored the role of the endocrine system, the impact of environmental factors on hormonal health, and the long-term strategies for sustaining testosterone levels. By understanding these dynamics, readers are empowered to make informed decisions about their health and take proactive steps to maintain optimal hormonal balance.

Throughout this book, we have underscored the significance of seeking guidance from healthcare professionals, as individual needs and responses may vary. Regular check-ups, hormone testing, and personalized treatment plans can provide invaluable support on the journey to hormonal optimization.

In conclusion, "The Alpha Formula" serves as a comprehensive guide to help men over 40 elevate their hormonal health and vitality. By implementing the strategies and habits outlined in this book, readers can take charge of their well-being, unlock their peak performance, and enjoy a fulfilling and vibrant life. Remember, the key lies in consistent commitment, informed choices, and a proactive approach to hormonal health. Here's to embracing the Alpha within and embracing a life of vitality and well-being.